*I'll Never
Be Fat
Again!*

Also by Carole Livingston

TO TURN YOU ON
WHY WAS I ADOPTED?

CAROLE LIVINGSTON

I'll Never Be Fat Again!

LYLE STUART INC. Secaucus, N.J.

First edition
Copyright © 1980 by Carole Livingston
All rights reserved.
Published by Lyle Stuart Inc.
    120 Enterprise Avenue, Secaucus, N.J. 07094
In Canada: General Publishing Co. Limited
    Don Mills, Ontario
Manufactured in the United States of America

Library of Congress Cataloging in Publication Data

Livingston, Carole.
    I'll never be fat again.

    Bibliography: p. 285
    1. Reducing—Psychological aspects.   2. Reducing.
I. Title.
RM222.2.L537   613.2'5'019   80-14661
ISBN 0-8184-0298-9

For L.

Without you there would be
nothing. You make it all
happen.

Acknowledgments

I want to thank the many people who helped with *I'll Never Be Fat Again*.

I'm especially grateful to Sandra Stuart, Arnold Levy, Irma Greenbaum and Sherry Armstrong for reading it in manuscript and making helpful suggestions.

Contents

Introduction

From time to time, people have commented with surprise on how thin I am—while at the same time I seem to be so busy eating everything in sight. I belong to the Wine and Food Society. I belong to the *Confrérie de la Chaîne des Rôtisseurs*. I belong to *Les Amis du Vin*.

I own at least fifty cookbooks and subscribe to many magazines published about cooking. My favorite program on television is *Julia Child & Company*.

Food? I go to the best resturants in the world. Last year I dined at least ten times at New York's Palace Restaurant (reputed to be not only the most expensive restaurant in the United States, but one of its best) where dinner is a four-hour affair. In Paris, I dine at three-star restaurants like Lassere (I'm a member of their Casserole Club) and Le Taillevent.

Many of my friends are food-conscious, too. This means feasts at their homes, and feasts in mine.

Recently I supervised an exotic dinner comprising twenty-five different delicacies for a group of more than one hundred guests.

Not long ago I was co-chairperson of an ice-cream tasting. The most highly praised ice creams from all over America were flown into New York so that members of the Wine and Food Society could sample twelve scrumptious tastes ranging from Graeter's chocolate chip from Cincinnati, to caramel cashew from Clancy Muldoon of Los Angeles.

I'm five feet four inches tall.

This morning I weighed myself.

I weigh 117 pounds.

I once weighed 162.

I'm not now the thinnest woman alive—nor was I the fattest.

But I'm thin and I like myself and I'll never be fat again.

Interested?

What You Will Find in This Book—and What You Won't

Would you like to know how I did it?

If you're an overweight person or even a person "on the brink" then I'm going to help you *if you want to help yourself*.

You've heard that song before. The reducing business is a huge one. There are whole industries that produce diets, diet books, diet candies, diet supplements, and diet gadgets.

Not many women's magazines would dare publish two consecutive issues without offering something in the way of weight-reducing advice. We're being bombarded with information all the time. Lack of information is not the problem. What is the problem is that few of us understand ourselves, and most of us don't understand our thorough involvement with food.

The key to it all is so simple that it just *seems* profound.

Recently, at lunch, I said something in passing to the editor of a national magazine. I hadn't meant to say anything momentous, but later she told me it had changed her life.

The topic of conversation was my history as a thin person after years of being a fat one.

I mentioned to her that at a certain point in my life I realized that in order to be slender I would have to give up something. I would have to overcome my childish instinct for instant gratification to obtain the larger gratification inherent in my becoming thin. Unbeknownst to me, this comment started her on a serious program of weight reduction.

A happy aftermath to the editor's story is that upon losing weight, she found her Prince Charming. But I don't want you to believe that the reward for being thin is romance. Rather, being thin contains its own satisfactions. You will like yourself thin. If someone else happens to like you, too—great!—that's a bonus.

If you have a weight problem, deep in your heart you've known the following for a long time: Being overweight is dangerous to your health. Extra pounds precipitate some illnesses and increase the propensity for others. Excess pounds shorten your probable lifespan.

But you've known this before I wrote it, and it hasn't stopped you from remaining fat, anymore than the sure knowledge of the dangers of cigarette smoking have stopped millions from continuing that slow-suicide habit.

The pleasure instinct is a strong one. So strong that we have a special word for an excess of it—hedonism. Sometimes the pleasure urge is so strong that it will lead people to such conscious self-destructive acts as the in-haling of "angel dust," the injection of heroin, or the abuse of the body with other dangerous drugs.

Some people literally eat themselves to death. I read recently about a woman who, while being carried by stretcher to a waiting ambulance, confessed that she had overdosed on Mounds candy bars!

An extreme case? Perhaps. But every overweight per-son has experienced overeating to the point of making themselves ill.

If you think the above example extreme, how about the fattest man in the world? There is a man who weighed 1,400 pounds. *1,400 pounds!* He went on a fast, but his body retained all fluids. In other words, he wasn't eliminating any waste. He was killing himself by dieting! The fire department's rescue squad had to remove a window of his house to get him out. They fashioned a stretcher of thick plywood to cart him to the hospital. At last report he had lost 900 pounds and was on his way down to normal weight.

But back to less excessive examples. Like you and me.

Body types are familiar to us all. Many books have charts to show you how much you should weigh for your height and frame. I know these intimately. When I was fat I always conveniently fit myself into the "large frame" category. Unfortunately, I never could manage to increase my height to adjust my actual weight to the "proper" one listed on the charts!

You are not going to find any such charts in this book. To paraphrase comedian Flip Wilson, you overweight people know who you are. Besides, don't we look at these charts trying to convince ourselves that we aren't as fat as we know we are?

In these pages, you also will not find recommendations to buy those frequently advertised gadgets that promise to determine the amount of excess fat you may have on your body.

One such device is a caliper that is used in the "pinch test." The pinch test measures the amount of fat in specific areas on the body, such as the back of the upper arm or a spot just above the hip. I'm not sure what you are supposed to learn after you've pinch-tested yourself. You may have the type of body that does not have a lot of fat in those particular areas. If that's the case and you "pass" the pinch test, does that mean you aren't fat?

I have never met a thin person who bought one of these things. Overweight people are the market. They are purchased more for reassurance that we aren't really overweight than for practical use. The fact again is people who buy them *know* they are fat. Do we all share a secret wish that one day, one of these gadgets will show us that we aren't fat?

To repeat: thin people don't buy them. As a matter of fact, *many thin people don't even own a scale!* How many overweight people can make that claim?

Don't you marvel at how fascinated we are with finding out *exactly* how much we weigh? Although it's not a gadget, there is a method of figuring out the overall proportion of fat to the rest of the weight of your body (your fat ratio). This is more accurate than height/weight charts, but not simple to determine.

Jack H. Wilmore, Ph.D., a professor of physical edu-

cation at the University of Arizona, tells us that we
start out at birth with ten to twelve percent body fat.
By the time we are in our early twenties, this has increased to fifteen percent for men and twenty-five percent for women. Because we eat too much and exercise
too little, we have a tendency to enlarge *both* our total
fat and the ratio of fat to the rest of our body weight.

If that's not discouraging enough, Dr. Wilmore points
out that on average, Americans gain "one pound of
weight a year after twenty-five—which adds up to thirty
additional pounds by age fifty-five."

Do you *really* want to figure out your fat percentage?
Then go to a sports physiology lab where they will
weigh you under water in a special tank. You are told
your total volume and, guess what? You can look up on
a table to find out what your fat percentage is!

You've now traded height/weight charts for fat percentage tables!

Where does this leave you? Still fat. You won't find
any recommendations here about finding out your fat
ratio.

What you *will* find is a sound, sensible, workable and
realistic approach to geting thin—*and staying there.*

It's the "staying there" that's important. Nay, *critical!*
If you're a dieting veteran, you know about the formerly
fat psychiatrist who became fat again. Or Johnny
Carson's sidekick, Ed McMahon, who is once again a
chubby.

This book is different. It reveals a successful approach
because I have been in your war, fought all the battles,
and I have won!

Unlike people who write diet books, I'm not going to load you with lists of specific foods to eat or not to eat. I'm not going to tell you when to eat your meals. I *am* going to share with you some vital concepts I have learned about reducing that will help you. I will share with you the ultimate secrets of becoming thin. *And I will tell you how to stay there.*

First of all, I'm lucky. Lucky because the first time I became aware of a need to reduce, I was only thirteen years old. You may wonder, "What's so lucky about that?" After all, many people spend their youth and many years beyond that totally unaware of what they put into their mouths. But I have observed that sooner— or later—even those people who have been "naturally thin" all their lives begin to put on weight.

Olympic gold medalist Peggy Fleming skated for more than 22 years and never thought twice about keeping her figure trim. She was surprised, therefore, after giving birth to her son, Andrew Thomas, that it took her a long time to get back into shape.

An exercise class helped her regain her lovely figure. She admits that now it is harder to stay thin. Her solution has been to eat five or six times a day—with each of those meals made up of very small portions of food. That, combined with running, does the trick. For Peggy Fleming, food-consciousness came at the age of 29. To her credit she learned how to handle it.

Since I became weight-conscious at an early age, I've had a lot more time to learn about reducing. I almost feel sorry for those who suddenly find themselves with more pounds than they'd like to be carrying and almost hopeless about what to do to get rid of them. For them it's more difficult. Not impossible—just more difficult.

But now I want to tell you my story.

Important: Throughout this book, there are chapters to which Intermission Exercises have been appended, and others which have lists to help you. If you really intend to get the most out of this book, please don't just turn pages. Don't pass by the Intermission Exercises or lists. Take the time to do the exercises and study the lists before going on to the next chapter. It won't take much time and these are designed to be truly helpful. You'll find your time is time well spent.

INTERMISSION EXERCISE

Sit still in a quiet place and think about *how* and *when* you got heavy and *why* you think you stay that way.

Do this for five uninterrupted minutes—by the clock.

My Story

I was the thin one in my family. Thin, that is, only by comparison. My father was six feet three inches tall. Tall, but not enough to justify the 240 pounds he usually weighed. My mother was only five feet tall. Most of the time she weighed in at 185. And my sister, at five feet seven inches, frequently carried well over 200 pounds.

With examples like them I didn't stand a chance.

As I said earlier, by the time I was thirteen, I was already chubby. Naturally, no one in my home took notice. But at school, where many of my friends were petite and slim, I became self-conscious. "Birds of a feather" frequently do flock together, and so I gravitated towards the other chubby girls with whom I could guiltlessly share the delights of the yummy chocolate iced cupcakes which happened to be a specialty at our school cafeteria.

A few years later, in high school, my main ambition was to become a cheerleader. By then I had accumulated more than just a few extra pounds. And thus came the first time when I had to face a dilemma I would encounter many more times in the future. I wanted to be a cheerleader. I also wanted to keep eating those cupcakes. I wasn't stupid. I knew I couldn't have my cupcakes and eat them, too.

I had to give up something—in order to obtain something else. And the something else was *very* important to me at that point in my life.

I want to repeat this because it is such a critical point:

I had to give up something in order to attain something more important to me.

I didn't give up right away. It seemed that no sooner had I conquered my chocolate-iced-cupcake craving, than something else equally tempting came into view. And along with that came the technique of finding someone who had the same problem. (Remember those same-feathered birds?)

In this instance both the temptation and technique were in one package. While many of my friends were slim and petite, Phyllis was not. She and I clung to each other like hot fudge clings to cold ice cream. A lot of the time, Phyllis and I complained to each other about our overweight. Much of the rest of our time was taken up feeding ourselves from the never-ending variety of freshly baked cookies that Phyllis' mother made in (I swear) ten-pound batches. When these ran low, we would slip into the dining room where six different kinds of candy were always available. These were piled high on a lazy Susan server which, when rotated, temptingly displayed the selections.

My favorite was, and still is, milk chocolate bark. If

you don't know what chocolate bark is, you are missing a taste treat. Simply described, it is chocolate candy with almonds throughout that is broken from a large "sheet" by the vendor. Not any of that fancy boxed stuff, this is candy for the hardcore aficionado.

Let us pause for a moment. Consider the above paragraph and note how vividly I still remember that chocolate bark. I was barely an adolescent when I first tasted it; it's years since I last tasted it, yet the taste memory clings to me.

I believed when I was trying to reduce, that once you got thin—*Vogue* thin—you never wanted those things that made you fat in the first place. Total victory would be mine, I thought, and I would never gaze longingly at a cream puff or a Malomar cookie again.

Well, let me tell you a truth. There *are* some foods that no longer have the same importance to me. I can, and quite comfortably do, live without them.

I know people who are really crazy about bread. Bread and I parted company (with a few exceptions) years ago. Sandwiches? I barely remember the last time I had one. Of course, take me to Paris where bread is not bread, but rather a taste treat not to be missed, and I eat bread.

What I'm saying about other foods that I love—and add pounds—is that I still crave them. I can still conjure up not only their images, but their taste as well. And, should I ever be locked in a room all by myself and someone slips a dish of chocolate bark under the door, you can bet that dish will be empty in a matter of minutes.

Temptation is *always* there. Those foods will always call to us. And sometimes we eat them.

What then is the difference in our behavior? Well, remember in the beginning of this chapter I said that I discovered that in order to attain something important I would have to give up something else? (In this case, the chocolate bark candy.)

The difference is not that I don't continue to want it. I do. The difference is that now I don't eat it most of the time.

I have a built-in scale in my body. This scale doesn't measure weight. It measures desire. It talks to me and I talk back. We have conversations all the time. Most of the time the dialogue goes something like this:

Me: "Wow! That lemon meringue pie looks delicious."

Scale: "Careful! You know what lemon meringue pie can do to your waistline."

Me: "Yes, but look at it! That meringue must be six inches high!"

Scale: "When was the last time you ate lemon meringue pie?"

Me: "About six years ago."

Scale: "How was it?"

Me: "Well . . . not so terrific. As a matter of fact, the crust turned out to be soggy. And the meringue only looked fluffy. It tased like soap bubbles. I think I got sick."

Scale: "Well, think it over."

Okay, I've exaggerated to make a point. In reality, however, I do *consciously* gauge how much I want a "forbidden" food against how much I'll have to pay for it. Payment, of course, is in pounds, not dollars. Much of the time I decide it just isn't worth the price. Sometimes I decide it is. *And then I eat it.* And I eat it without any guilt at all. Because *I* have made the decision. *The food hasn't decided for me.*

This brings me to a word I just used that I want to reclaim. "Forbidden." When we reach the point of making conscious decisions about what we eat, there aren't any forbidden foods.

Dr. Nevin Scrimshaw, head of nutrition and food science at Massachusetts Institute of Technology, concurs. He points out that "There is no such thing as a 'fattening' food—any food eaten to caloric excess (when we consume more calories than we expend as energy) will make us gain weight."

You may substitute my word "forbidden" for Dr. Scrimshaw's "fattening." Keeping those two words in mind, remember too that the foods we select and the way we prepare them has a lot to do with the number of calories we consume. Rather than banishing the food from our diet, we must learn to forbid ourselves to prepare these foods in ways that will put more pounds on our bodies.

For instance—what about potatoes? Ahh! Remember potatoes? Most dieters avoid them like botulism. They *are* fattening, right? Wrong! That fact is, potatoes are fairly *low* in calories and are a pretty good source of vitamin C. But . . . if you slice them and fry them in oil, they become French fries; when you mash them with butter and milk, they become mashed potatoes. Get the message? Obviously, it is what we add to the potato that makes the calorie count shoot up. Potatoes in and of themselves have an undeserved bad reputation.

Another "forbidden"food to most dieters is pasta. Would it surprise you to discover that you can eat more pasta than French fried potatoes for fewer calories and have a good protein source at the same time?

All dieters could benefit from a quickie course in food values and nutrition. Our ideas would change about what is "forbidden" and what isn't. Again: *It's what we do to food and how much of it we eat that adds the fat, not the food itself.*

I want to say something more about what we can now refer to as non-forbidden foods and about conscious decisions.

If I could relive those days I spent with Phyllis and the cookies and the lazy Susan bearing candy and put my current attitudes into action here's what would happen.

I'd look at the cookies and the candy and think about them. I would try (though not always successfully) not to eat them without being aware of the pleasure that I wanted to derive from the experience. After all, what's the point of eating only to nourish a guilty conscience? I would thoroughly enjoy a selection of cookies—making sure I had at least one of each kind.

I would then turn to the candy and very possibly eat more than I intended of the chocolate bark. But this time I would probably skip the gumdrops and spice drops. I've discovered that I don't really love them all that much. And I hate the way they cling to my teeth, making work and money for my dentist.

Do you get the point?

The important difference in my eating pattern today is that I now eat *by selection*. Selection is when *you* make the decision that you really do in fact want a specific food. You have thought about it for a while (this can be seconds, minutes, hours, even days) and you have concluded that eating it is worthwhile; even though it may mean skipping something else.

Here's an example of what I do. Not long ago I located a bakery that makes one thing better than any other bakery I have ever found: giant chocolate chip cookies. (In case you haven't figured it out by now, I am a great fan of things chocolate!) I really love these cookies. It takes quite a bit of effort for me to get to the bakery since it is not near my home. So . . . when I decide that I have to have a chocolate chip cookie, I think about it and plan for it. And when I get it—I consume it with total pleasure.

There is almost a ritual attached to it. Since I know I am going to eat it and want to enjoy it thoroughly, I make sure to pick a time when I can accomplish that. It's usually around 9:00 P.M. when I'm ready for my evening mug of tea. That's also when my daughter, Jenny, is asleep. That way there's no chance of her trying to get any of my cookie. This is *not* a sharing moment. It's a time I reserve for my own personal indulgence.

Selfish?

Sure. But I believe we are all entitled to some things in life that don't have to be shared with others.

When you get to the point of planning to have some favorite item, go ahead. Enjoy it.

When I make this decision I am *never* guilty about eating. When I eat without thought, I suffer acutely. Because for me, guilt usually drives me further into unconscious eating. And that's a tough cycle to break.

Tough, but not impossible. The noted psychologist, Dr. Albert Ellis, points out that *now* is the time to break the cycle. Not at the end of the day or week or month. The moment you find yourself bingeing is the time to get control. Who ever set the arbitrary rule that Monday or the first of the month or New Year's Day or the first of July was the time to begin diets? Any minute of any hour of any day is the time to stop bingeing. And don't waste time berating yourself for having fallen off the wagon. Just get back on! I guarantee you that you'll feel good about yourself for having stopped the binge.

But back to my story.

INTERMISSION EXERCISE

Think about one food that you have always considered forbidden—because you believe it makes you fat. Make sure it is something you really crave.

The next time you want it, promise yourself to wait ten minutes (by the clock) before eating it.

After ten minutes, ask yourself again if you really want to eat it. If the answer is yes, go ahead—and enjoy it.

If the answer is no—you have just taken one giant step forward. You have made your own decision. *The food has not decided for you.*

Congratulations!

My Family

As mentioned before, my entire family was fat. And not just by a few pounds. I mean *really* fat. My sister, Jane, who was two years my elder, was always seriously overweight. Even as a child I remember seeing how she suffered the taunts and teasing of children her own age because of her size.

One day I asked my mother when Jane first became fat. She told me it was after she'd had her appendix removed. Hearing that explanation, I thereafter associated appendectomies with getting heavy. Not until many years later did I discover that Jane had her appendix removed when she was five years old! I suppose my family wanted to believe it was the operation that caused her to gain weight. It probably made them feel less guilty about her being heavy at a time in her life when she could have little responsibility for it.

I am intense about the subject of children and weight. Watching Jane spend a tortured childhood (that is not an exaggeration—because children can be cruel to each other when they find even the smallest flaw) is perhaps one of my most vivid memories. As a girl, Jane could only shop in the "chubbies" department. Later it was into half sizes. When she did manage to lose some weight, she could never keep it off.

My parents don't deserve all the blame. As an adult, it was Jane who kept herself fat. However, my folks obviously didn't teach either of us proper eating habits. In that way they certainly helped keep her heavy, and started me on the road to having a weight problem.

When Jane and I were children, chubby babies were considered cute. People believed skinny kids were unhealthy. This is a concept that exists in other countries up until today. In Greece, a person who has an enormous belly signifies someone who has a lot to eat—and thus a person to be admired. There the average weight—especially of women and children—is between 12 and 16 pounds heavier than the European and American average. Fatness and appetite are associated with good health.

This distorted idea arose in Greece from many years of food shortages. For example, during World War II, several hundred thousand Greeks died of starvation. It's no surprise that heavy eating became associated with life and with health. Now, however, the Greek nation is campaigning to make people aware that obesity is a negative goal.

Awareness of the dangers of obesity has increased. Medical researchers have concluded that the number of fat cells we have is determined at childhood. Once you have more fat cells than normal, the best you can hope to do is to keep them at a normal size. Unfortunately, people with more fat cells than normal will always have more difficulty reducing.

Parents have a responsibility to educate their children about the benefits of good-eating habits. If they do a good job, their kids may never need a diet book.

How can parents prevent children from becoming obese? For one thing, they can stop interpreting feeding as a demonstration of love. In some cultures, food is so entwined with the concept of giving and receiving love that to refuse to eat is interpreted as an outright rejection of the person offering the food.

Another step parents can take is to stop using food as a reward or as a pacifier. It's very simple to program children to overeat. Dr. Hilde Bruch, a psychiatrist at the Baylor University School of Medicine in Houston, Texas, says, "All the mother has to do is give the child food whenever he cries, no matter what the reason for the distress, or not feed him when he's hungry because it's not yet time to eat again."

What then happens is that the child will have no will power. His brain will never learn to distinguish hunger from being bored, feeling depressed or disappointed. And he will have one reaction to all of these feelings: he will eat.

Instead, feed children when they are hungry rather than on a specific schedule—and don't make them eat if they are not hungry.

I am determined that my daughter will not have a

weight problem, at least not of my doing. I have had to unlearn many of the habits I learned as a child in order to help Jenny grow up thin. I consciously stop urging her to "Eat" and, instead, I watch her appetite patterns. The fact is, she has a very small appetite. Instead of filling her plate with food that she will leave (and aggravate me), I give her tiny portions. If she wants more, she asks for it. If she doesn't, I accept her decision that she has had enough.

Observe your children. As infants they instinctively stop eating when they are full. But even as five and six year olds, they start to take on the habits we have taught them—and overeat. If you make your children believe that cleaning their plates makes you happy, why, that's just what they'll do. They'll try to please you, and that's not the purpose of eating.

It's difficult to look at a baby in a crib and conceive that you are presenting that child with an emotional problem by overfeeding it. As that infant grows into a chubby toddler, a stout youngster, and a chunky teenager, it will put on a thick suit of emotional armor needed for self-protection.

The child may act happy because this is one way to defend oneself from hurtful comments, ridicule and feeling bad about one's image.

Unlike that age-old notion, fat people are not jolly. Oh, they may act jolly, but as Jane used to confess, "What else can I do? Should I cry when people make fun of me?"

Rather than cry, many fat people pretend they don't care about the ribbing they take. And they usually do a convincing job. That's because fat people are treated as if they were a separate race.

Even alcoholics usually evoke more sympathy than fat people. Being fat is an undeniable admission that you can't control yourself. And, to most of the world, overeating shows a childish lack of self-control.

Losing control by overeating isn't any worse than losing control by drinking too much. But socially it creates a great deal of prejudice against the obese person. The alcoholic can hide his problem for a while, but let's face it, fat people stand out because their problem shows.

Sure, it's unfair, but that's the way things are.

There have been attempts to organize fat people to convince themselves and others that they are content being fat. Let them come up with all the zippy slogans they want, I will never be convinced that fat people are happy about their size.

I do believe that fat people suffer mightily.

If there's a case for being fat, I won't present it. This is a book to help you to lose weight—not to make you feel great about being heavy. However, having watched Jane grow up very heavy and suffer because of it, I am sympathetic to the emotional plight of obese people.

One in a while Jane managed to slim down for a short period. She was very pretty. I know what you are thinking . . . but Jane *was* pretty.

Unfortunately, there was not enough motivation going for her to stay thin. And inevitably, the pounds would creep back onto her. Later, as a young adult she married a rather thin fellow. If it was not tragic, it would have been comical because of the obvious Jack Spratt comparison. Jane's husband liked her being fat. Well, it's not that he liked her fat, but as I have discovered about many relationships, as long as she stayed fat, he felt less threatened about losing her affection. Whenever she tried to reduce, he worried that she would become attractive to other men and then, he'd risk losing her.

I'm sure you've encountered situations like that. In such cases, you've got the thin one mouthing weight-reduction encouragement, even while subtly sabotaging the reducing program.

"Aw, go on, honey, it won't hurt just this once to have a piece of the chocolate cake. You can go back on the diet tomorrow."

If it isn't a spouse who sabotages you, it may be a "friend." I deliberately put that word in quotation marks because sometimes it is not until you try to reduce that you discover who your friends really are.

One woman I know has lost nearly 80 pounds after being heavy most of her life. She is shocked by how many of her "friends" have been cautioning her against losing too much. They tell her, "Now Sherry, don't get too thin." Or, I'm sure you have heard about those "friends" who tell you how bad or ill or haggard you look as you reduce.

Apparently, our associates are frequently more comfortable seeing us as we have always presented ourselves. That way we are not threatening them or their conception of us. They can have compassion about their poor, fat friend who just can't help being that way.

As the saying goes, with friends like that, you don't need enemies!

I wish Jane's story had a happy ending but it doesn't. She died at the age of 32 from a ruptured cerebral aneurysm. Because she had been severely overweight most of her life and had suffered from high blood pressure, her entire body was under tremendous stress. Although physicians say aneurysms are congenital, you can't convince me that her obesity did not contribute to her death.

I wish I could brighten my story here, but I must make my point in order for you to understand what did and did not motivate me in my determination to stay thin for life.

To continue the family story—my father, as I mentioned earlier, was also very heavy. (By the way, when I say *very* heavy, I am not talking about ten or twenty, or even thirty pounds overweight. I mean much more than that. He was obese.) He, too, suffered from high blood pressure. At the age of fifty-one he, quite suddenly, suffered a fatal heart attack.

My mother, another victim of high blood pressure (don't forget she was barely five feet tall and averaged 185 pounds), suffered a number of strokes. At the age of sixty, she was more like eighty years old. She entered a nursing home, hardly able to walk and with severely impaired speech. Two years later she died of a ruptured abdominal aorta.

Wow!

I must admit, every time I think about it, the whole

picture staggers me. It is quite obvious to me that because my family was chronically obese, they were prone to many illnesses they might have avoided otherwise.

Most of us are aware of the connection between obesity and certain illnesses. Experts keep reminding us. Dr. Theodore B. Van Itallie, director of the Obesity Research Center at St. Luke's Hospital Center in New York City, reports that "In countries where people tend to be fat, there is more endometrial and breast cancer—as well as more atherosclerosis, blood lipid disorders, strokes, heart attacks, gout, and gall bladder disease."

The strongest connections are between obesity and hypertension and adult-onset diabetes. I don't know if my family was fortunate that it wasn't prone to diabetes; maybe they just didn't live long enough to get it!

The conclusion is obvious: Obesity can kill.

That fact scares me. And my family history scares me even more.

Whenever I have a headache—which is quite rare now that I'm thin (I used to suffer from them frequently when I was heavy)—I immediately wonder if I'm next. If my blood pressure is slightly elevated, I become concerned.

I wish I could say that all this is why I decided to be thin, but that isn't the truth. The family story is an afterword to my own experience. And part of the reason I have described it is to illustrate a point: People do not reduce because of fear.

People don't get thin because they're afraid they're going to die.

Of course there are exceptions. People frequently *do*

lose weight *after* they have had a heart attack and their doctor tells them if they don't get thinner, they will have another one. People go on diets when their blood pressure goes up, but most return to eating as usual once their pressure returns to normal.

You see, secretly we all believe we are immortal. We tell ourselves: "Everyone else may die, but death will somehow pass me by and *I* am going to live forever."

Absurd? Put down this book and think about it for a minute. Isn't it true that although rationally you know you are going to die, deep in your heart, you don't really believe it?

Sounds crazy, doesn't it? Well, psychiatrists tell us it's a universal craziness. Crazy or not, most people go through life believing "It won't happen to me." To other people, yes—but "Not to me."

Keep in mind that *you* are somebody else's "other people"!

Well, if fear was not the motivating factor for me, what was?

And, on this cliffhanger, let's pause for a moment.

INTERMISSION EXERCISE

Mentally draw your family's physical (health) profile.

Are you the exception, or are other members of your family also overweight?

Has any one of them ever reduced—and stayed thin?

Why and How I First Lost Weight—or, How to Stop Kidding Yourself

What is the strongest motivation for becoming thin? Obviously, this isn't a question that can be answered easily. And the answer will differ for each person. But you can find similarities among people and with that in mind, let's continue.

On a short-term basis, a strong motivating force can be a particular goal. In my case, the first time I lost weight was when I wanted to become a cheerleader. I went on a crash diet, lost about fifteen pounds, and made the squad. I didn't stay thin for long. Once secure, I went back to the cupcakes and managed to stay on the cheering squad, too—a bit heavy in the thigh, but a cheerleader still.

My second short-term goal was getting in shape for my wedding. Actually, it was the need to fit into a borrowed wedding gown. The gown was quite beautiful, but the only way the endless row of buttons would close was if I got rid of about twelve pounds. I made it.

If I didn't have to return the wedding dress—or perhaps if I wore it daily—I might have kept the weight off. However, during the first year of my marriage, I discovered the joy of freshly baked apple pie and gourmet cooking and 11:00 P.M. coffee and cake.

I gained twenty pounds. Of course my husband also gained twenty pounds, so who noticed? Moreover, it seemed to me that everyone around us was heavy.

At that time I never thought of myself or of my friends as heavy. Looking back, I can't believe the amount of food I consumed. Perhaps people were not as weight-conscious in the 1950's and '60's as they are now. At least my circle of friends was not.

If a woman wore a size twelve dress, she didn't consider herself stout. Today, fashion has accustomed us to dress sizes that top off at ten. On the down side you can even find women putting on size twos. (Is anyone *really* a size two?) And have you noticed how a new size is appearing in the shops marked "extra-small"?

Frankly, I wonder if designers don't just label clothing with sizes smaller than they really are. They understand the psychology of female shoppers. Most women would be thrilled to fit into a smaller size than they thought they needed. I know that the first time I fit into a pair of pants marked six, I ran with my money to the cash register. I didn't care whether or not they looked good—they were a size six! And that meant I was skinny. I wouldn't be at all surprised if clothing was soon marked "small," "extra small" and "teeny-weeny."

Not everyone overweight admits to being uncomfortable about it.

Recently a publication appeared speaking for fat people. The magazine called *Big Beautiful Woman* is the result of its editor, Carol Shaw, being unable to find attractive clothing for her stout figure. She uses the term "fat" with no apologies. Though we may not all look like movie stars, Ms. Shaw stresses that "everyone—no matter what size she wears—is entitled to the most up-to-the minute, fashionable clothes available."

Ms. Shaw started her magazine when she became angry at the lack of appealing apparel for heavy people. While she does not promote fatness, she does advocate ending discrimination against fat people—especially women.

We have reached the point where our bones must be barely covered with flesh or much clothing we see for sale will not fit. Even the "roomy" things don't look good unless you are very thin. We are obviously manipulated by fashion towards slimmer and slimmer figures no matter how we try to keep our weight goals realistic.

Let me illustrate—using women's fashion again, since it changes so drastically.

I don't know if you were around when skirts were tight and belts were tighter. I had a very wide leather belt that had a spiral closure. Once it was on, you needed to turn the spiral ever more tightly until you could barely breathe.

We used to push ourselves into skintight jeans and then stand in the shower wearing them. After they dried they were even tighter. Pants were so slim that sometimes they had zippers at the ankle to allow you to get into them.

Time passed and fashion changed. Clothing got more comfortable and skirts weren't tight and pants had nice wide legs—and even pleats at the waist—so that the size tens and twelves could occasionally fit into a smaller size.

More time passed and, as you can probably guess, we were back to tight jeans and skinny skirts. The pendulum continues to swing back and forth from tight to roomy to tight.

If you don't like what they are showing you don't have much of a choice because all of last year's fashions always manage to disappear each new season. And we model ourselves after the ultra-skinny mannequins who show off the new styles.

It's no surprise that we demand a thinner profile of ourselves than we did in years gone by. Now we want the clothing to look as good on us as it does on the models. I have concluded that I am now about as thin as I can get without fasting every other day. (This is quite different than the rationalizing I used to do when I was reducing. Then I used to believe I would faint if I didn't eat something every four hours. Or, I'd have headaches every time I started a diet.)

Years later, after I had reached my goal, I was sure that most of the symptoms people describe when they begin dieting were imagined. They were rationalizations, just like mine. All excuses to avoid dieting.

Imagine my surprise to learn that headaches *are* common at the beginning of a diet. That's right, you're not making it up after all, and neither was I.

A panel of physicians specializing in weight reduction was queried by the editors of *Obesity/Bariatric Medicine* magazine. The consensus agreed that many people *do* suffer headaches when they begin reducing. There are several causes, including emotional ones.

Emotionally-based headaches are the result of using food as a pacifier. There are also metabolic causes for headaches, such as low blood sugar (mild hypoglycemia) which is caused by the reduction in carbohydrates the body is taking in as compared to before the diet.

Sometimes, with the reduction of carbohydrates, the dieter experiences a sudden and severe diuretic effect. That's when the body loses a great deal of fluid. You know, when you're in the bathroom all the time. With the loss of fluids you can also lose sodium and potassium (one of the problems with the protein sparing fast that was popular recently).

I could describe clinically and graphically what happens to the blood vessels in your head, but it's sufficient to say you end up with one whopping headache.

Whatever the cause, emotional or physical, it's a real headache you may be suffering. But hold up before you feel vindicated about abandoning all attempts at reducing because you can't bear the headaches. Keep reading.

These same physicians agree that the headaches are only *temporary*. You might want to take an aspirin or Tylenol to relieve the symptoms. Or, if your headache is caused by low blood sugar, a teaspoonful of honey or small glass of fruit juice will do the trick. Properly treated, your headache will disappear within a few hours, or days.

Just as headaches can be real, so may be your problem of putting on the brakes when you have reached your goal.

I realize that if you are considerably overweight as you read this it may be difficult to consider the danger of going too far in the quest to become thin. Ironically, however, *compulsive eaters tend to become compulsive dieters,* and your goal should be to achieve a realistic weight and stay there—not to reduce to stringbean size.

An extreme example of compulsive under-eating is the disease anorexia nervosa which is getting a lot of attention these days. The literal definition of anorexia nervosa is an hysterical aversion toward food.

Here you are, reading a book that will help you reduce, and now I'm telling you about people who can't stand food. However, this disease is as dangerous in its way as excessive weight is in its. Usually young girls around puberty are the victims. They starve themselves because they can't be convinced that they're thin.

They frequently look like concentration camp prisoners, having reduced to virtual skin and bones. The result can be (and often is) fatal. Treatment for this disease is difficult because the victims can pretend to eat and then rush to the bathroom to vomit it all out. Or, they take overdoses of laxatives to pass food through their digestive system too rapidly. Hospitalization and psychiatric care are usually advised.

Sometimes young college women who want to lose

weight fall into a pattern of starvation, binge eating, and vomiting. The technical name for this is bulimarexia. And if you think it's rare, psychologists in New York's Cornell University believe that as many as one-quarter of Cornell's freshmen may be afflicted.

You may wonder if I have gone off the track a bit. But this book is not only about reducing, it's about learning how to deal with reality about your food intake.

How many times have you starved all day because a party was scheduled for that evening and you wanted to be able to "enjoy yourself" without restriction? And how often does that plan explode in your face when you get to the party so famished that you have no control and thus eat everything served that isn't gray or nailed down?

It is better to get into the habit of eating something —a piece of cheese, fruit, almost anything—to take the edge off that starvation feeling. Use this same principle whether it's a party or an intimate dinner at a friend's house. By eating something before arriving at the party or at your friend's house you will be able to eat from choice. The few calories you consume in this exercise will actually prevent you from eating out of control.

I am reminded of a memoir written by a Prussian nobleman based on his life. Married to a Spanish aristocrat before World War I, Baron Paul von Zglinitski and his wife would heat frankfurters over their candlestick chandeliers. Dressed in tuxedo and evening gown, they would eat these before going to the affair of the evening. At the party, they would eat like mice: just little nibbles. This was the aristocratic way!

My book is concerned with taking weight off and keeping it off—in a healthy way. It's designed to teach yourself and your children good eating habits so that neither you nor they end up obese *or* anorectic.

I want you to lose all the weight you feel you should. You can learn to be sensible about food and not become undernourished. If you don't take precautions to eat foods that satisfy your hunger and keep your body in good health, you may find yourself thin, to be sure, but not feeling good.

Perhaps some of those people who provoke the comments about how bad they look thin may actually look bad, because besides limiting their calories, they may have also been shorting their bodies of vitamins, minerals, and the rest of the ingredients that keep human beings alive and healthy.

If your reducing progam is sensible, you will look better as you reduce than when you were heavy. You can't cheat your body; the outside will reflect what's going on inside, for better or worse.

I make this point because there is a strong case to be made for the fact that although Americans may be eating less, they are ignoring nutrition. Moreover, as if things weren't bad enough, they are not necessarily losing weight.

We've become a nation of lazy people. D. Mark Hegsted, administrator of the U.S. Agriculture Department's Human Nutrition Center, observes that Americans are more sedentary than ever.

In spite of the popularity of jogging these days, jogging isn't the total answer. If you have a job where you find yourself sitting all the time, jogging simply cannot make up for the lack of overall exercise. The dieter's tendency is to decrease even further the number of calories to try to compensate. It doesn't work.

Keep in mind when you are being realistic about your weight goal that when you reduce your caloric intake, you may, as Hegsted points out, also find you are not consuming the recommended minimum daily amount of nutrients. While your calorie needs decrease when you reduce, your nutritional needs do not.

I will show you how to discover when you've reached that realistic weight goal. Once you're there I want you to be content with your weight, as I am.

I am happy with the way I look and feel. I don't want to go without eating—so this is it for me. But it wasn't always that way.

After my first year of marriage and the addition of those twenty pounds, I found myself lumbering along. I'm the type of person who gets heavy all over so I convinced myself I wasn't heavy just because my employer teased me by saying he heard me clomping down the hall.

I found myself wearing a lot of basic black. Coco Chanel once sold fat people on the idea that the color black is slimming. Look around and you'll see a lot of large people dressed in black. (Believe me, they are not all in mourning.)

I also wore pleated skirts because some fashion authority once said that pleats hide fat. If anything, they emphasize it. You have to be very thin to wear a pleated skirt because the pleats are supposed to lie flat, not bulge the way they did on me.

Well, the high point for me (or low point, depending on your point of view) followed my first trip to Europe. In three whirlwind weeks, I gained fifteen pounds. I was eating constantly, and enjoying every mouthful. Each new city brought new taste delights. And I was determined not to miss anything. I don't think I did.

When I returned home, I was the fattest I had ever been! I could no longer ignore it. Nothing fit me. When I went shopping for new clothes, I couldn't believe the sizes sales ladies brought out. They couldn't be offering these to me? But they were.

I was genuinely upset. For the first time in months, I examined myself closely. I looked in the mirror. Dr. Arnold Wechsler, author of *The New You Diet*, suggests we all look in our mirrors. "If you are satisfied with what you see, don't diet," he advises.

I was *not* satisfied with my image. No matter how hard I held in my stomach, it still hung out. My thighs were chafed from rubbing against each other. My pants were worn out in the spots my thighs rubbed. My wedding ring was tight. *My shoes were tight!* (I went down an entire shoe size when I got thin!) Yecch! I hated myself.

I did the only reasonable thing under the circumstances. I went on an incredible eating binge. To soothe my hurt feelings about discovering the fat girl who stared at me every time I looked in the mirror, I ate more.

To add insult to injury, when I asked my husband if he thought I was too heavy, his response was not the one I looked for. (Naturally, I wanted him to be the mirror on the wall to my Snow White.) A bit reluctantly, but truthfully, he told me, "Well, to be perfectly honest, you are putting on weight."

That blunt answer supplied all the motivation I needed. My binge ended. Since my husband was also somewhat portly by then, we decided to diet together. This was very helpful because we gave each other moral support. If someone works with you, it can be an important factor for success.

We turned to Weight Watchers.

INTERMISSION EXERCISE

Two questions to ask yourself:

1. When was the last time you went on a crash diet so that you could fit into a special outfit or because you were going on vacation and wanted to look good in a swimsuit?

2. After the vacation was over, did you keep your weight down?

Weight Watchers—and Other Things to Watch

At the Weight Watchers meetings I saw people who made me look like a toothpick, but I wasn't turned away for being underweight. We were all accepted.

We shared our stories and applauded each other's efforts. I heard more rationalizing about not being able to diet than I thought existed. Some pleaded that "the holidays are coming"—meaning they couldn't consider dieting for the period beginning with Thanksgiving through Christmas and New Year's and with very little effort you could stretch this on to Arbor Day.

Others said they couldn't possibly live without bread. Or pasta. Or mashed potatoes. All excuses. We found we *could* live without these foods and we *would* live without them.

(By the way, today the Weight Watchers' menu has been expanded to include many of the foods which were excluded when I was on the program.)

49

I threw myself totally into the program and went through Thanksgiving, Christmas, and New Year's successfully. As a matter of fact, I could have been up to my nose in cranberry sauce, but I wouldn't have eaten any of it to save my life.

I found the motivation of the group and the steady weight loss so reinforcing that I got more pleasure out of being able to say "no" when offered food not on my program, than I would have had in eating it.

Although I was successful in reducing during the holiday season, this is an exception to the rule. I would advise you to be tolerant about your cravings during such times.

If your attitude is to *maintain* rather than lose weight during the holidays, you can face the New Year with renewed vigor towards your reducing program.

Eventually, I lost twenty pounds and reached "goal." I will forever be indebted to Weight Watchers for helping me.

I continued dieting long after leaving Weight Watchers, not because I was dissatisfied, but because their "goal" was just more weight than I wanted to carry.

I learned much about eating nutritiously from Weight Watchers. However, I also discovered a serious flaw in their program.

A Weight Watcher feels safety in the knowledge that there are some foods which can be eaten on an unlimited basis. These are the variety that don't add any weight and may even be negative foods. (Radishes are an example. The red radish burns up more calories to digest than it adds to your caloric intake.)

It's helpful to know that in an emergency—when you feel you must have food in your mouth—there are foods you can eat "legally." If you follow the advice I offer though, as you reach your weight goal, you will not only become a thinner person, you will also become a person who is in control of your food management.

You will discover that no matter how "legal" a food may be, there simply are times to eat and times not to eat. One of the keys to staying thin is managing this balance. By the time you finish this book you, and not your fork, will control when you eat.

The Carole Livingston approach will transform you from a person who thinks "fat" into one who thinks "thin."

Let me clarify this concept. When I was heavy—and even after I had lost those first twenty pounds—I felt secure knowing that if I got desperate I could eat some things in quantities to pacify me. In those days I still believed I was a fat person *lucky* to be temporarily thin. I knew that eventually I would get fat again. I always did. Most serious dieters are like this. As a matter of fact, like clockwork, every year (usually at the same time) they begin their diet. Then, they gradually put it all on again. And the following year, right on schedule, begins the diet.

At that point in my life I kept all my "fat" clothing because I knew I would need it, sooner or later.

Later—much later—I learned that when I truly believed I was thin I didn't need the security blanket effect of having food around so that I could eat all the time. I *could* do *without* food for a period of time. I *wasn't*

going to faint if I skipped lunch. I learned self-control.
(Remember that concept? When we are infants we have
to learn self-control in toilet training, in not shouting
out in class, etc.)

If we merely substitute "good" foods for "bad" ones,
we haven't yet learned that there are decisions to make
about eating or not eating.

One of the reasons we stay fat is because we continue
to cling to that infant-like belief that we just can't stop
ourselves. That means you can eat and blame yourself,
forgive and go on eating because you have condemned
yourself as weak-willed and a baby.

Overeaters can also blame "outside influences" for
eating foods in quantities they later regret. I used to do
it all the time. For example, I traveled to work by subway. I took the same train to work in the morning and
the same train home at night. Routine. But if anything
disturbed that routine I would use it as an excuse to eat
something I shouldn't. If the train was late, I "rewarded"
myself for waiting. After all, it wasn't me who made the
train late, so didn't I deserve some goody?

Sound familiar?

An important part of being thin is *accepting the responsibility that you make yourself the way you are.*

If you are fat, you made yourself that way. If you are
thin, you made yourself that way, too. *Nobody else did
it to you!*

Very simple—but a very difficult concept to truly
understand and make a part of yourself. I know this be-

cause it took many years for me to understand it. After reading this, you'll be able to benefit from my experience and embrace this concept now.

When I accepted responsibility for eating or not eating, I no longer rewarded myself for late subway trains. On the contrary, I found myself passing up foods that I knew would make me fat. My reward was in the knowledge that I could wait until I was able to eat to my satisfaction.

I was proud of passing up these foods. I sympathized with those who made excuses, as I used to, about why they got fat again. "My mother insisted that I eat everything on the plate." "If it's there, I eat it." "If I don't eat it I'll hurt his/her feelings," etc., etc.

There's that infant attitude again. Getting fat is out of your control; it's something other people or outside forces do *to* you.

Stop kidding yourself. We do it to ourselves. Whenever someone tells me they can only diet if everyone around them helps out, I know that person is not accepting the respsonsibility for making his or her own decisions about food.

Taking this responsibility is not easy. (I never promised you it would be easy!) In fact, it's *very* difficult. But it is possible to accomplish. Only *you* put the food into your body and only *you* can prevent it from entering. You make all the decisions. Once you accept this, you have taken an important step forward.

Before telling you about my next step, let me suggest your first steps.

FIVE STEPS TO GET READY:

1. Get a notebook. This will become your food diary as described later in this book.

2. Mark the first page "Past" and describe your own history of overweight. When did you begin to get fat? Why did you begin to get fat?

3. Mark the second page "Present" and record the ways in which you are keeping yourself fat. List all the foods that you can recall eating during the past twenty-four hours. List all the foods you eat today that are between-meal snacks.

4. Mark the third page "Future" and write down all the reasons why you want to become a thin person. (Not just "get thin" but *become* thin—and stay thin.)

5. Turn to page four. Record two numbers. One will be your accurate weight today. The second number will reflect the number of pounds you'd like to weigh one year from today.

Now put away the notebook and read on . . .

Liking Myself
(the Vanity Syndrome)

It seems simple now, looking back, but it took a while for the vanity syndrome to work for me. For quite some time after I lost weight I did not give up my "fat" wardrobe.

Holding on to the "fat clothes" was the same as holding on to the belief that inevitably I would get fat again. However, the longer I remained thin—and got even thinner—the more I liked myself. It was also true that I felt better, but it was the image in the mirror that really turned me on.

My weight loss was achieved in stages. They weren't planned stages. However, since they were gradual it gave me a chance to become accustomed to the constantly changing me. Whenever I reached a plateau and couldn't get any thinner, *I concentrated instead on staying at that weight.* As long as I didn't put on any weight, I was temporarily satisfied.

What I was not prepared to do at that time was to give up a number of foods that kept unwanted pounds on me. Compared to the "old" me, I was skinny. So I stayed slightly overweight for a long time.

Speaking of plateaus, have you ever wondered why two people who appear to be eating the same number of calories don't always lose at the same rate? Generally the heavier you are, the more weight you will lose. Some people, however, do lose faster than others. And men lose weight with more ease than do women.

This has nothing to do with liberation, ladies! It's biology. The Associated Press reported on research done at the Medical University of South Carolina where twenty-two men and eighteen women were studied for twelve weeks. On average, men lost fourteen pounds while women only took off seven. (The men started out averaging a weight of 230 against 176 for the women.)

Why? Well, the research team points out that "The body composition of males contains proportionally more muscle and less fat than that of females." Translated: men lose more rapidly.

If you keep that in mind, you'll never go on a weight loss bet with a man. And, you may have found at least one answer for an occasional plateau you reach, while the guy next door doesn't.

There were positive aspects of my plateaus. Although I wasn't as thin as I am now, I *was* learning to feel good about myself and my figure. And this helped build my self-esteem.

You can use a plateau positively to prepare yourself for the time that you will again feel ready to reduce.

Although part of this is rationalizing, part is being realistic. It's especially difficult to reduce if you are not positively motivated. As long as you promise to get back to the diet—maybe even by setting a date on your calendar—you will stay on a forward path.

My next dramatic weight drop was a positive side benefit of illness. Others have told me of similar situations. For instance, a good friend confided that although she had always been stout, during a brief illness she lost a great deal of weight. After that, a very unhappy personal crisis caused her literally to lose her appetite. Her depression was so severe that she simply couldn't eat.

I've heard people say, "When I'm depressed, all I can do is eat." That's the case for many overweight people. But at moments of true despair, appetite often does disappear.

After her depression lifted, my friend decided to enjoy the ironic benefits of her misfortune. To this day she has kept her trim figure.

I do *not* recommend depression or deliberately getting ill as a realistic weight control device. I hope this is clear! If you find yourself thinner after being ill or glum, your body will probably need the nourishment it couldn't accept while you were sick in order to keep you healthy. Don't—I repeat, don't—go searching for a mild case of anything!

My illness happened to be a bad back. I found myself bedridden. For three weeks I was permitted to get out of bed only once a day.

I panicked. I was certain that having nothing to do all day but lie inactive in bed, I would again grow fat.

I was so upset by this possibility that I became compulsive about not eating any more than I normally would. As a matter of fact, I tried to eat less to compensate for lack of exercise. Unwittingly, I began using many excellent devices to stay thin and I've since learned these are often used by successful dieters.

Each morning, before my husband left the house, he brought to the bedroom, where I lay, all the food I would consume during the time he was away. I had a cozy little setup at my side, with a toaster oven, Thermos jug of coffee and so forth all within arm's reach.

Since I could not get out of bed, I ate only those foods that had been prepared ahead of time. I knew in advance what I was going to consume. I use this same principle successfully now. Planning what you will eat before you eat it, helps to cut down on unconscious overeating.

At the end of my bedridden three weeks, I stepped on a scale and was astonished. I had lost five pounds! This proved to me that you don't have to gain weight when your daily routine is disrupted. Disruption is a great excuse—but only for those seeking excuses to fatten up. (Remember I learned *not* to reward myself with food when the subway train came late.)

I learned that I really did have control over myself and I justifiably felt proud.

It would have been easy to say, "Well, I was in bed for three weeks and put on a little weight."

Who would blame me? Who would not sympathize with a bedridden person? But who is it you are trying to convince that you've done the right thing? Yourself, that's who. Instead of making excuses, I had turned my illness into a triumph.

By the way, before you get the idea that I have a will of iron, let me confess that along with self-control, I understood that I would be very depressed if I got fat while in bed. So I was protecting my emotional well-being as well as my figure.

As time passed, I began to replace my out-dated "fat" wardrobe with new clothing. I symbolically let go of my fat image by letting go of those clothes. With my new figure, I wanted to reward myself—but this time it was with pretty things instead of with food.

As I shopped I was conscious of the considerable cost of buying new things. This pushed me into a syndrome that acted to motivate me further. If I was going to invest in a new wardrobe, I couldn't afford to replace it if I got fat again. Thus, more and more I found myself committed to my new figure.

The next stage in my weight loss occurred during and after pregnancy.

Once again, I was filled with anxiety about gaining extra pounds. I'd heard stories about women who had been skinny all their lives until they became pregnant— and then, the cravings were just too strong. One woman told me that during the last four weeks before giving birth, she did nothing all day but sit in front of her open refrigerator and eat.

Was I going to go the same route? I remembered those three weeks when I'd been bedridden with my back

injury. If I didn't use that experience as an excuse to get
fat, I decided I couldn't use pregnancy either. Pregnancy, after all, is not a disease. Frankly, I never felt
better in my life. I kept my weight gain within the limits
suggested by my obstetrician and after Jennifer was
born, I not only returned to my normal figure but
dropped a few pounds to boot.

I reached the conclusion that just because some
women get heavy during pregnancy, and stay that way
later, doesn't mean that they all do. And I wasn't going
to be one who did. By the way, you might look around
and notice lots of women with children who are not fat.
They obviously got through it successfully too. Others
simply "use" pregnancy as the excuse to gain. ("Hey,
I'm going to be looking fat anyway, so what's the difference if I go crazy and eat more?")

The next period of my weight loss is most interesting
and familiar to all of us. I wasn't ill, pregnant, or even
very much overweight any longer. I was at that point
many of you may recognize. I only wanted to lose another ten pounds.

After those ten pounds, I promised, I would be happy.
Then I would never have to go on another diet for the
rest of my life.

Here, by the way, is a time during which dieting *can*
become compulsive. Particularly if you're not very clear
about your goals. The closer you get to your goal the
more you may try to reduce just a little bit more, "for
security." I found that when I lost even one "security"
pound, I immediately considered this my new weight

level. What had been intended as an extra pound *under* my ideal weight, so that I might be able to overeat once in a while, quickly became absorbed in my thinking as my new ideal weight.

You will learn, as I did, to keep to your goal and not strive to reduce below it. Otherwise you are toying with compulsive dieting.

When I set about losing those last ten pounds, I was going through a divorce. (I guess you *could* say that when my husband and I parted I lost 185 pounds!)

There was no special drama connected to the dissolution of my marriage that sent me into the depths of depression. On the contrary, I found myself freed from schedules, especially those that meant I had to prepare breakfast, lunch, or dinner. Except for my toddler, I didn't have to cook meals if I didn't want them. And, I could eat what I wanted, when I wanted to. By this time I virtually had memorized calorie charts and knew what I should eat. I also had learned (thanks to Weight Watchers) a balanced approach to eating.

I decided to eat *only if I was hungry* and then, I would eat practically the same thing for every dinner. (I hadn't read about one-sided diets then. I had simply devised my own.)

Oh, there was a short period after the divorce when I ate on the run, or spooned tuna fish right out of the can in order to save washing dishes. However, after a while I found myself getting depressed. It didn't take long to realize the depression was because I had turned dinner from what should have been a pleasant experience into something mechanical and boring. For me this meant that eventually I would become careless about what I ate and that would mean trouble.

I deliberately changed my eating patterns. After all, wasn't I worth having dinner with? I liked myself and decided to treat myself that way. And so, every evening, at dinnertime (I use dinnertime as an example because I was away from home at work during the day), I would set the table for myself. I used a place mat and napkin— a real cloth napkin, not paper.

If I was having wine with my meal it wasn't in a grape jelly glass; it was in the best wine goblet I owned. Sometimes I ate by candlelight. And whether it was steak or hamburger, I sat down and enjoyed it. I ate my dinner at an hour when my daughter was happily occupied or, if that was not possible—and sometimes with children it certainly is not—I waited until she was asleep.

My attitude was totally pleasure-oriented. I made up my mind that if I was going to eat, I was going to enjoy it.

Before very long I had dropped those ten pounds.

You may have noticed that throughout my story about losing weight, I haven't been very specific about what foods I ate or did not eat. I haven't told you what to eat or when. If I did that, this would be just another diet book. It isn't. Anyway, by this time in your dieting history you've undoubtedly read all about green leafy vegetables and the like. You know what you can and can't eat. And you also know that some things work for some people and some don't.

There is no diet, no form of weight reduction that will

work for everybody, all of the time. That is why I could not successfully go back to Weight Watchers to lose more, even though it had worked for me once.

There is no magic, no pill you can swallow at night and wake up lighter the following morning (no matter how we wish otherwise, me included). And it's *never* easy. No matter what any book ever tells you, if they say it's easy, drop it like a hot 93-calorie potato.

Why do you think so many diet books are best sellers? They are bought by the same group of people—those perennial seekers of the magical weight-loss sceret.

Save your money. This could be the last weight-reducing book you will ever need. Once you have made your decision to become thin—and stay thin—the next step is to realize that, simple though it sounds, it isn't going to be easy.

Yet, if you can channel the energy you once spent on buying pastry into feeling good about the change in yourself, you can be one of a very elite group. You may become one of the fewer than ten percent who reduce and continue to stay thin. Fewer than ten percent? A depressing statistic? *Not if you are determined to be one of us!*

Time to ask yourself once again: "Do I sincerely want to become thin and stay thin?"

If that answer is "YES!"—let's move along. Let's examine some positive and negative approaches to taking it off.

Getting Ready

The first step in losing weight isn't to read all the diet books you can find. It isn't going to the doctor. It isn't filling your house with low calorie beverages and throwing out all the pretzels.

The first step is admitting to yourself that you *need* to reduce.

I have met many people who look at me like they are in urgent need of cottage cheese and celery but you couldn't convince them. Somehow they ignore the expansion of their waistline and the need for extra holes in their belts. By the way, I'm not talking about a few pounds overweight, I mean h-e-a-v-y.

So, first of all, admit that the dry cleaner isn't shrinking all your clothing, which I once believed had happened to me. It was during a trip to Paris, after I'd spilled perfume on the trousers of one of my suits. Off it went to the dry cleaner. On getting the suit back, I was absolutely flabbergasted. Trying to get the pants on,

I could not believe that the cleaner had not shrunk them. I pulled them off quicker than a wink and didn't dare to try them on for a long time.

A few months later (and a few pounds lighter) I casually pulled on the same pants. Not so magically, they fit. It was me, not the dry cleaner.

Dry cleaning *can* temporarily make some clothing seem smaller. But that's only temporary. Don't kid yourself. It is your body that is expanding—not your clothes that are shrinking.

The next step in getting ready to reduce is to decide not to indulge in self-pity about admitting to yourself that it is, indeed, necessary to reduce.

Self-pity is similar to hating yourself for being out of control. It only leads to food binges. Then you enter into a cycle that is difficult to break. Besides, self-pity is simply another method we all occasionally use to delay getting on with what we really want to do.

Okay—you've admitted you need to lose weight. And, you did manage to throw away part (if only a sliver) of that candy bar instead of devouring it entirely. Great! You're back on the track. Now for the next step.

This step is an important one. It's when you must decide that today is really the day you are going to begin.

Really today.

Not a week from next Wednesday. Today!

Now. *This minute!*

I hear the voices already . . . "But I have to decide which diet to choose." "I have to shop for the 'right' food."

Sure, you will need to do all that. But you can do it even while you take your first step to the goal of a thinner you.

Impossible? Not at all. You aren't going to pass out if you miss a meal because you don't have the "proper" food in the house. (If you recall, I thought that would happen to me. I'm here to tell you it won't.) Honest. And among the foods already in the house, I'll bet you can find something "right" to eat even while you are making your plan.

I have almost never been in the house of an overweight person where there wasn't a container of cottage cheese in the fridge. True, it frequently goes from purchase date to mold formation without being touched. But it's there. If it's still edible, eat it. If not, there's got to be something non-fattening to eat.

More important than what you are going to eat for your next meal—you have made a giant leap towards becoming thin!

TWO WAYS TO STRENGTHEN YOUR RESOLVE:

1. Say out loud, "Today is going to be *the* day I am going to change my eating habits forever." Do this before each meal.

2. The first time today that you're tempted to eat something you know you shouldn't eat, go into a different room and say out loud: "I don't need this food. I'm going to trade it off for my long term goal."

Planning

You've taken the step. Congratulations! What you have accomplished by deciding to get thin—for the last time—is to take your life in your own hands. You have made the decision to have control over food and not the other way round.

The decision alone should make you feel exhilarated.

The fact is, at this point, you actually haven't *done* a thing. But do you notice that you feel a sense of accomplishment? That's because *you* are the boss now. There are few feelings that can beat this one.

I know this feeling so intimately that I want to pause here to assure you that I *do* understand what you are going through. I know that whenever my weight begins to creep up I have to go through the very exercise I've just described. I call it "collecting myself," just as a rider collects his horse before starting out.

Here's something you can try right this minute.

69

Stretch up tall. When you walk, walk tall. You will feel better. Fat people slouch, thin ones don't. Start thinking thin.

I have taken a great deal of time describing "getting ready" because if you are not ready, nothing is going to work. If you *are* ready, just about anything will work.

It's that basic.

Okay, so you're ready. Now what do you do?

I would suggest that you make an appointment with a physician for a thorough examination. This can never hurt. It also costs money, and for some people financial involvement is an important incentive toward weight reduction.

When you see your doctor, tell him that you plan to lose weight. After he stops applauding, he may make some helpful suggestions. He may even hand you one of those mimeographed diet sheets we have all been given at one time or another. Remember, though, don't wait for your appointment. That's just another delaying tactic. Today is the day, right? Right!

The fact is there really isn't any special preparation for dieting once you make a decision to do it. You can do it this minute. Recall my description of being a Weight Watcher during the Thanksgiving and Christmas holiday seasons. Remember, too, that I was so positively motivated that exposure to many tempting foods didn't make me eat them.

The next suggestion is to read up on nutrition. The last time I had to learn about nutrition was in Montauk Junior High School hygiene class.

There are any number of sources of information.

Adele Davis is one of the best-known names in the field. Dr. David Reuben has written *Everything You Always Wanted to Know About Nutrition*, which may help you. Or you can write to the Food and Nutrition Information and Education Resources Center (FNIERC) for its free catalog that lists more books and other literature available about food than you ever dreamed about. FNIERC's address is Room 304, Beltsville, Maryland 20705.

Your local public library also has a variety of books on the topic. If you are going to lose weight effectively, you owe it to yourself to learn what protein, vitamins, minerals, carbohydrates, etc., mean to your body.

You don't have the time? You're in a hurry to get on with it? If you've taken the time to invest in this book, don't stop at this point. Remember, your goal is to become aware of what it is that makes you fat. One step towards awareness is learning how the food you put into your body reacts once digested.

Planning helped me enormously. Whether you have a hundred pounds to lose or only a few, a plan is essential.

Have you consulted the charts? When I was heavy I always considered myself "big boned" so that I could fit into the "large frame" category. Even if I was wearing panties and a bra when I stepped on the scale, I always allowed myself two pounds for clothing.

If I could only have grown taller, all my problems would have been solved. After all, I was about the right weight for a woman of five feet ten inches tall. Now that I'm slim I realize that those charts can be a joke. They merely act as a crutch to lean on.

When I got thin I never looked at a chart again. You *know* you're thin when you are. You can see it in the mirror. Charts are for people who want to convince themselves that they are not as fat as they know they are. Knowing you're thin is like knowing you've had an orgasm; if you only hope you've had one, you haven't. It's something you can't mistake. You can't make a mistake about being thin either.

Okay, so you have told your physician about your plan to reduce. You're going to become an expert on food values. Now tell your family and friends.

Tell your father, your mother, your mate, your co-workers, your dog. Tell everyone. Why? For one thing, you'll want to have them on your side. For another, the more people you tell, the more committed you will be. You don't want to humiliate yourself in front of everybody by failing, do you?

Through it all you'll avoid being hurt by lack of interest by others if you recognize the fact that your dieting may be a compelling matter for you, but is not always of that much interest to the people around you.

Obviously, it's more important not to forget your promise to yourself. But let's be realistic. You want to have as much going for you as possible. Look at losing weight as a sort of war—and in war you use every weapon you can get your hands on.

I'm also a person who benefits from sharing information. I guess that's why Weight Watchers succeeded for me. Organized groups of dieters such as Weight Watchers and Overeaters Anonymous are effective partly because people share each other's dilemma. It works because you admit that you need their help, and it makes the group feel good because you believe it can help. Also you can profit from learning by example. Everybody is working together.

Recently Weight Watchers has combined the group help concept with summer camp. Ordinarily, we think of children when we conjure up the image of camp. And Weight Watchers has had camps for some time for youngsters who want to lose weight. But now adults have the opportunity to go to camp, too. Thus, you can enjoy the atmosphere of summer camp, while at the same time, working seriously on losing weight.

The atmosphere is not that of a luxurious spa. Rather, there is a sense of "roughing" it, a definite plus for many of the "campers" who shy away from glamorous spas as too posh for their taste.

There is a sense of work to be done by most of the participants who, as of this writing, pay approximately $400 for a week's stay. (The rates decrease the longer a camper remains, although the average stay is two weeks.)

While there is an ambitious program of activities offered each day including stretching exercises, arts and crafts or nature walks, tennis, swimming, and so forth, no one is forced into any of these. Indeed, as one camper reported, some people do little more than make it once around the campus.

There are Weight Watchers camps for both adults and children in many parts of the country. You can check with your local Weight Watchers for more information.

Such a program is particularly appealing to those who are positively motivated to reduce by sharing their problems with others. This method will not work for everyone.

If you are the type of person who will not benefit by sharing your weight reduction plans with others erase everything you have just read from your mind.

This book is about helping you to get thin. No single approach will work for everyone. I want you to get thin. I'm flexible too. I am the first to admit the use of many approaches to keep trim, sometimes changing from one day to the next.

Do not tell anyone (except maybe your doctor) that you are on a diet. This might sound like an about-face but it really isn't.

I only advise sharing if you believe it will help you get thin. For those who will *not* benefit from this, I will have lots of other ideas for you. For you sharers, stick with me as I continue a while longer in discussing the benefits of this approach.

Now that you are publicly committed to dieting and your family and friends are put on notice (and have been reassured that you are serious about this) you can start to plan.

By the way, when you announce you're going to lose weight and you hear collective groans and know they are silently asking "Again?" don't be discouraged. Admit to them that, "Yes," this is another—yet another—attempt to reduce. But this time you are going to do it until you get it right! If you can convince them that you need their help, they may stop groaning and start assisting. (However, as I suggested earlier, beware of diet saboteurs!)

Although I don't usually recommend negative rein-forcement, this is war, as I said. Leaving yourself open to your friends' jibes and teasing when they catch you cheating can present quite a challenge. You are on the spot to prove to them (and to yourself) that you can stay on the straight and narrow. In any event, the win-ner will be you as the pounds come off.

Back to planning.

Now is a good time to decide how much weight you want to lose. What is your goal? Is it realistic? I mean, if you are a woman who is six feet tall, it's not very realistic to believe you can ever reach 100 pounds—and stay alive. But then again, why would you want to?

If you are a male six-footer, don't shoot for 135 as a realistic goal. You can discuss goals with your physician. Or, if you must, go ahead and consult a height and weight chart. Get an image of what you want to look like.

Close your eyes and picture yourself thin.

The next step is to decide how long it will take.

Stop now and think about all the crash diets you have been on. Obviously, in the long pull they don't work or you wouldn't be reading this.

Don't be in a hurry at this point. This planning step is a crucial part of your weight-reduction program. Being sensible about how much you want to lose and how long you expect it to take is critical.

You must be realistic. Remember, you are now ready to give up the belief in magic pills and formulas. You didn't get fat overnight, so it's silly to believe you can take it off that way. (Read this paragraph a second time. Before you have finished reading this book, you will understand that it is a key to the ultimate secret of successful weight loss.)

There's another one of those deceptively simple sentences. You can read it and think you understand it. Take a moment now to digest the significance of what you've just read.

All right—you've decided that today is the day. You've told everybody about your decision (or you haven't, if you are the keep-it-to-yourself type). You've set a realistic goal and determined how long it's going to take. Now for the next step.

INTERMISSION EXERCISE

As part of your reducing program, read at least one item about nutrition. Whether it's a chapter in a book or an article in a magazine, promise yourself to learn something that you didn't know before about food and how it is used by your body.

What Works and What Doesn't—Sometimes...

What are you going to eat? What are you *not* going to eat? When, where, how are you going to eat? Don't panic. Let me tell you some of the things that helped me and some that helped other people. Let me also tell you some things that don't help. And let me repeat: nothing will work for everybody all of the time. And— IT'S NEVER EASY.

In the last chapter I devoted a lot of space to the "sharing" approach. I also allowed for those of you for whom that is the worst piece of advice. Perhaps you need to keep your diet to yourself. Maybe you couldn't bear to watch your friends anticipate another failure. (Or, perhaps you lack self esteem and enjoy the humiliation that fat and failure bring!)

What is most important is to *understand your needs* and to devise an approach that will work for you. It might be fun to surprise people with your weight loss.

Obviously, those who see you frequently will notice after a while that you are reducing. They may ask if you are on a diet.

You can have some fun by pretending that you didn't even notice that your clothes are starting to hang on you. They'll think you have suddenly become a guru about eating, having quite unconsciously discovered the secret of true thin bliss.

If that turns you on, go with it. But be true to yourself and keep on the right path.

As we all know, some people will do *anything* to lose weight. Lots of people pay large sums of money to go places where they don't eat anything. Fast farms. They go into seclusion.

In upstate New York there are many of these "fast" farms where people sit around and ingest nothing but water. The proprietor of the most widely known one admitted to me that she could never have made it so big were it not for the repeat business.

Men and women have been known to drop as many as fifteen pounds in three or four days at a fast farm. Then they leave and often, in a day or two, put it all back on. A psychiatrist friend says that what happens is that the body becomes anxiety-ridden by the sudden weight loss and can't wait to recover the weight. Thus her insistence that the only lasting way is a gradual loss.

Some people insist that they need an initial jolt to change their direction and an immediate loss to encourage them. In that case, fasting on a limited and carefully supervised basis can be helpful when you begin a new diet program. However, what many of these people don't want to accept is that at some point you are going to have to leave the fast farm and face the world of food again. Your scale may reflect an encouraging weight loss, but if you are not prepared to follow up with a practical approach to eating, you will be back in the same spot again before very long.

The same philosophy applies to any program that isolates you from the world.

Recently, a newspaper editor with a weight problem went to Duke University in North Carolina where they specialize in helping obese people reduce. When last reported (after a stay of several months) he had reduced by more than 150 pounds! However, if he doesn't change the way he eats, which made him fat in the first place, he will certainly put the weight on again.

Lyle Stuart, the publisher for whom I'm writing this book, is a classic example of the "successful" faster who failed. Some years ago, he discovered the protein-sparing fast. He drove four hours for his first visit to the doctor who was administering it. Lyle wouldn't wait for the week necessary for the doctor to study the medical test results: he insisted on going on the protein-sparing fast that day. *Immediately!*

Lyle Stuart is a strong personality and the doctor couldn't resist his demand. The doctor put Lyle on the fast at once.

For 120 days Lyle didn't swallow anything but water, a pink protein liquid, and some vitamin tablets. During this time, he took groups of people to the finest res-

taurants in Paris and New York. He hosted banquets at
his fabulous home in Port Maria, Jamaica. And while
his guests feasted, he fasted, showing off by sipping his
pink liquid.

Some people marveled at his determination. Others
cautioned him with "If you don't eat, you'll die!" or tried
to discourage him with, "You look terrible."

Actually, he looked different—but he looked marvelous.

As a result of his personal experience, he persuaded
the doctor to produce a book called *The Last Chance
Diet*. It was an immediate best seller. It became the diet
book of the year, in time selling more than two million
copies in all American editions. It was published in
Germany. It was published in Holland.

And Stuart himself? After 120 days, he lost 83 pounds.
Eighty-three pounds in 120 days! Incredible. He flew to
Rome and had his tailor, Angelo, make a complete new
wardrobe for him. He stood at his company's exhibit
booth at the American Booksellers Convention in Chi-
cago, displaying himself in front of a poster of the old,
fat Lyle Stuart.

He had gone from 240 to 157 pounds.

There was only one thing wrong. True, the compulsive
eater had become a compulsive non-eater. But now the
fast was over. He'd reached goal.

Lyle Stuart broke his fast at a bookseller's convention
party where lots of Mexican food was being served.
Guacamole and chili and enchiladas.

He loved 'em. He'd always loved 'em.

So he ate. And ate. And the next afternoon he returned to the same hotel suite, where they were again offering Mexican food, and he ate and ate and ate.

You see, nothing had changed. His eating habits were no different than they had been before the fast. They'd merely been frozen. And now when they defrosted, he did what he'd always done.

He ate.

Today? Well, I can tell you that he has a closet full of never-worn elegantly tailored custom-made suits by Angelo of Rome.

Crash diets don't work except temporarily. Drastic weight loss will be followed by drastic weight gain.

The unhappy fact is that most people find they not only gain back *all* the weight they have lost, but many add a few pounds as topping.

Even more discouraging for the crash dieter is the phenomenon that occurs with subsequent attempts using the same crash method. The fact is, your body doesn't know how much of its fat is "good" and how much is "bad." And being a pretty intricate unit, it does its best to try to hold on to all of itself. It becomes thrifty. It manifests that thriftiness by developing a resistance to the same crash methods. Each time you try the same crash diet it will work less and less effectively.

One woman, who had crash dieted away eleven pounds in one week, found that, a few months later, using the same diet, she could take off only five. Her body had become thrifty. That doesn't happen when you reduce slowly and sensibly.

You don't really want to establish crash dieting as a way of life, do you? Be realistic this time.

Many people who can afford it go to lavish spas where they can be massaged and pampered while taking off unwanted pounds.

At the Golden Door, located in southern California, you can buy the luxury of being one of only thirty guests where eighty-seven staffers attend to your every need. The owner, Deborah Szekely Mazzanti, in her book, *Secrets of the Golden Door,* has described her life's work as the desire "to see that my guests carry home the conviction and the know-how to live and to grow with more life, for more years."

Many celebrities seek sanctuary at such places as the Golden Door or La Costa (another spa, also in southern California). Barbara Howar, television personality and novelist, goes regularly. She once told *Harper's Bazaar,* "I'm so relaxed when I get back, it takes about six months to start screaming at the children."

The total environment is appealing, and the food in very low calorie portions is beautifully served.

Such spas do indeed sound attractive. But there's a clue to the "lasting effect of spas" in Barbara Howar's comment, "All I really need is *one* more 'pit stop' a year at the Golden Door."

You might look upon visits to spas as luxurious vacations, for that is the category in which they deserve to be placed. Even if you could afford a La Costa or a Golden Door or other spas, the time comes when you must leave. Then you have to face reality and make food decisions on your own. So enjoy the spas, but don't think of them as a solution to staying thin.

INTERMISSION EXERCISE

Ask yourself: "Am I willing to accept the reality that losing weight is not easy?"

Are you finally willing to accept the fact that there are no miracles that will make you thin?

Take an honest inventory of all the dreams, wishes and desires related to the idea of miraculous weight loss.

Reveal to yourself these self-defeating illusions, and then move past them into the reality of a daily weight loss and maintenance program.

Diets! Diets! Diets!

The protein-sparing fast Lyle Stuart tried was developed some years ago in research directed by Dr. George Blackburn, associate professor of surgery at the Harvard Medical School.

Lyle Stuart's experience doesn't mean that the protein-sparing fast isn't effective. In can be, under controlled circumstances. Dr. Blackburn, together with Dr. Peter G. Lindner of South Gate, California, ran a program that involved 167 grossly obese patients. When it ended, Blackburn reported that eighty percent of his patients had been successful in reducing their weight; the average loss was 40 pounds, and those who followed the basic rules of the program stayed trim for the year or more they were monitored by watchful physicians.

The important ingredient that accounts for the success of these patients, and that was lacking for Lyle Stuart, was behavior modification. Without it, almost all of the people would regain the weight. With it, they were able to learn how to stay thin. Again, *they had to change their eating habits* on a long-term basis, not a temporary one.

Unless you decide to work closely with your physician, or nutrition counselor, don't consider this program. A further caution is that the protein-sparing fast is not a diet for people who have less than twenty pounds to lose.

I add that last comment because you may be thinking the same thing that I thought on hearing of the diet. At the time I had five pounds to lose and thought I'd go on the modified fast and drop them quickly. I'd not have to be concerned about planning my foods, etc. Did it work? Not for me. I simply didn't have enough weight to lose.

Which brings me back to my often-repeated point: not every diet will work for everyone.

In describing the protein-sparing fast I emphasize the inclusion of behavior modification, if the weight is to stay off.

Behavior modification is one of the most important concepts in weight reduction success. As most of us know (because we've done it lots of times), it may not be easy to lose weight; but it's even more difficult to keep it off. Actually, behavior modification is merely a new name for what people have done for years. Whether you call it relearning, re-education, changing your habits —it all adds up to altering the eating habits that made you fat.

First, of course, you do have to get the weight off.

Since we know by now that each person will respond differently to each approach, it's important that you find the way of reducing that you can live with. There's no point in eating grapefruit and peanuts for three months (sure, you can reduce that way, if you don't eat anything else) if you are not prepared to eat that way for the rest of your life. You must examine your current eating habits to discover how to design an approach to weight control that will be effective and realistic.

After pioneering the protein-sparing fast, Dr. Blackburn more recently climbed onto the calorie-control bandwagon as the "best" way to take off weight. In an article published in *Family Circle* magazine (November 20, 1979), Dr. Blackburn joined forces with Ruth A. Clark, R.D., a staff project dietitian with the Department of Dietetics at New England Deaconess Hospital.

Dr. Blackburn and Ms. Clark do not compare this program to the protein-sparing fast regime. However, the conclusion Dr. Blackburn has drawn after years of experience is that "a *diet* alone is not enough. . . . To be successful with *permanent* weight control, you must invest some time and energy in understanding *how, why, when, where* and *with whom* foods are eaten."

In the *Family Circle* article a choice is offered the dieter from seven food lists: I—Milk; II—Complex Carbohydrates (grains, legumes, pasta, starchy vegetables); III—Fruits; IV—Low-Calorie Vegetables; V—Medium-Calorie Vegetables; VI—Protein (fish, poultry, meats, eggs, cheese); VII—Fats (spreads, salad dressings).

The point of this approach is to avoid the boredom of dieting by *choosing* foods from the above categories. In other words, the calories are already counted for you.

Boredom is the major ingredient in most of the one-sided diets. Whether it's protein-sparing, any single food diets such as eating hard-boiled eggs, or rice, or bananas, or grapefruit, you frequently lose weight because you quickly become accustomed to the regimen and aren't particularly interested in overeating when you are limited to the few foods the diet allows.

A big problem of one-sided diets is poor nutrition. Though you may be losing weight, you may not be eating well enough to provide your body with the day-to-day vitamins and minerals it requires to keep you in good health.

The most impractical feature of one-sided diets is that they are aberrations. You aren't going to eat in that way for the rest of your life. So once the diet is over, you go back to old eating patterns and get fat again.

One-sided diets are all too often crash diets, and we know now that these not only don't work, but work less and less each time you try!

Some eating approaches aim at both reducing and good health. Certainly with the introduction of so-called natural and unrefined foods, more people are genuinely interested in combining weight loss with a healthy outlook.

Suddenly we started to hear about fiber. If you didn't include fiber in your diet, you were on the wrong track. Bran as a fiber source started selling like crazy.

What *is* fiber?

Well, the definition of fiber may depend on who is doing the defining. Traditionally, fiber is the leftover part of a food after it has been treated with chemicals that are similar to those which are involved in digestion. Or, to put it more simply, fiber (or dietary fiber, which is the term used these days by nutritionists) is the portion of the food we eat that is not digested.

With people now worried about dying of cancer and heart damage, there's strong appeal to a food, whose increased quantity in our diet could aid to prevent such illnesses as well as diseases involving the lower intestinal tract.

Fiber is discussed in an article in *Redbook*'s issue of January, 1977. Fiber may be linked to the advice our grandmothers gave to eat an apple a day to keep the doctor away.

Well, fiber is a bit more complicated than that, but essentially it entails adding bulk to the diet. Since so much food we buy is refined practically to the state of mush, bulk, if you want it, has to be added back.

According to the *Redbook* article, fiber does two things —first, it absorbs water in the intestinal tract and causes you to have a bulky and soft bowel movement; second, because the contents of your digestive tract are now bulkier, your excretions are speeded up. That's why fiber (such as bran) has a laxative effect.

If you believe the theory that the longer food stays in the bowel, the greater your chances for getting diseases like cancer, you'll think fiber is great. Get all that stuff out quickly.

What is the appeal of fiber for us dieters? Those who praise its use feel it encourages weight loss. As *Redbook* says, "Foods with a high fiber content require more chewing. And a high fiber content may inhibit absorption of nutrients through the intestines."

I'm not altogether convinced this helps you to lose weight. Maybe because fiber is bulkier you feel fuller. And, if you feel fuller, you may eat less. And, if you eat less . . . well, you finish the sentence.

Some of the over-the-counter diet aids produce a full feeling in the stomach, with the promise that this will discourage eating. It would appear that using fiber to give a bloaty feeling is not a new idea.

Scientists are naturally skeptical. Some caution against too much fiber in the diet, especially if you have colitis or diverticulitis. Surely fiber would aggravate these conditions. On the other hand, since we eat so many processed foods and refined grains, maybe we could add a little fiber to our diets.

Those who are in favor say it's difficult to eat too much fiber. Because you do feel fuller when you add bulk to your meals, you'll just stop eating when you have that bloated feeling. Obviously, this ignores the fact that most overweight people eat well past the point where they feel full. That's why they *are* fat!

If I seem ambivalent about fiber, it's simply because I've seen too many fads capture us and then pass away with little or no long range positive effect.

To be certain, once we heard about bran, it swept over us the way fibers are supposed to sweep through our intestines. One doctor quoted in *Redbook* referred to fiber as the "cholesterol of the '70s," and the *Wall Street Journal* reported that "because of this publicity, there is a shortage of bran on the market."

Imagine! A shortage of bran. Why, you probably couldn't give it away during the years before we started to hear about its "miracle" qualities. And that's what every fat person is looking for—a miracle. Something that will replace his own effort in reducing, something *else* that will cause you to drop weight without having to go hungry or feel deprived.

I don't really want to burst your balloons, but I do want to help you become an aware human being who won't always be a sucker for the next "cure" to come along.

Try fiber if you like. But don't expect to get suddenly thin because you are adding it to your diet. Add it but stick to whatever method you use to reduce.

Whether you attempt the protein-sparing fast, try Dr. Blackburn's latest calorie-controlled approach, or add fiber to your diet, the important point to keep in mind is, once you are thin, you must learn how to stay thin. And be assured that this book will help you, if you want to be helped.

Getting thin is only Act One.

My first success came through Weight Watchers. This works for lots of people and may work for you. A similar group approach is used by Overeaters Anonymous. There is a sharing of experiences and information and an extensive support system for people who admit they have a compulsive eating problem.

Overeaters Anonymous (or O.A.) does not prescribe specific foods to eat. Rather, they try to help members discover what drives them to eat compulsively. Like Alcoholics Anonymous, they employ a sponsor relationship in which members can call upon one another for support when they feel they are about to go out of control.

Many members feel that they have found people who understand their eating problems at O.A. meetings. Some have said that even their families, who try to understand their overeating, can't compare to fellow members who truly know what it means to go wild with food and who have experienced anxiety so unbearable that all they can do is think of eating.

If you think Overeaters Anonymous might be right for you, check your local telephone directory to see where there is a branch. The organization is non-profit and has been very effective for those who pledge themselves.

After completing the Weight Watchers program, I found it difficult to return to that method later on in life when I wanted to lose more weight. I no longer got as turned on by the group approach as I had earlier. By the way, this is not the case for everyone so I don't mean to discourage you if you are a veteran Weight Watcher and want to return.

I consider myself a successful Weight Watcher because I will always carry with me many concepts I learned under that program.

I also tried fasting and for a while this worked. I ate moderately all week long and then let loose ever the weekend. Desserts are my passion, so, from Friday night until Sunday night I allowed myself anything I wanted.

I must admit that this program was fun. At least for a while. I'd indulge all my sweet-tooth desires: cookies, cakes, muffins. I had it all. But on Sunday night it all had to go. Ironically, it all went, right into me. It never occurred to me that I could have thrown the uneaten goodies away! Of course, more often than not, there weren't any leftovers.

On Monday morning, all the cakes and munchies were gone and I would fast all day. (I later named this approach to maintaining my weight the "feast or fast" method. By the way, pay attention to the word "maintain" because that's what you do: you manage to keep to one weight. This doesn't get you thin.)

Fasting wasn't difficult after eating a large quantity of sweet foods. I was so bloated on Monday mornings I had little appetite. More, I usually had a rotten taste in my mouth and felt physically under par too. That discouraged eating. Years later I recognized that I apparently was reacting negatively to all those sugar-laden foods.

What I was experiencing, without realizing it, were food hangovers, triggered largely by the abundance of sweets I had eaten.

If you want to learn more about the effects of sugar on the body, read the book *Sugar Blues* written by William Dufty. Dufty, who was really obese, met Gloria Swanson. She converted him to a healthful diet. He became thin and the contrast was so great that old friends literally didn't recognize him on meeting him! He married Gloria Swanson.

If you find yourself reacting oddly when you eat sweets, it may be that sugar and you are not meant for each other.

Today we are starting to understand that sugar can not

only make you fat, it can make you ill. We observe the
behavioral changes in children after they have consumed
large amounts of empty-calorie foods loaded with sugar.
But in the past, if ignorance was not exactly bliss, it
kept me sweets-satisfied.

I managed to keep my weight pretty much at the level
I wanted it. For a while. Before very long, though, I
found it becoming more and more difficult to discipline
myself and Mondays would occasionally slip by without
fasting. The dial on the scale started to move up. I had
to change my behavior pattern unless I was prepared
to get fat again.

I changed.

Uppers and Lowers

Maybe you have thought about taking diet pills. There is a man I know who had been heavy most of his life. He went to a doctor who prescribed diet pills. The pills we are talking about are all variations of amphetamines—sometimes called "speed" or "uppers."

Amphetamines must be very carefully administered by a physician to avoid addiction. Not only is a tolerance built up by the body, meaning that larger and larger doses are required to do the job of curbing appetite, but it's also very difficult to stop using them as they're addictive.

Doctors who casually prescribe amphetamines have been dubbed "Dr. Feelgoods." The reason is obvious— amphetamines give you a feeling of euphoria. It's not easy to stop taking a pill that makes you feel good.

For most people this is a very dangerous way to lose weight. In fact, the government has taken steps to ban

95

the use of amphetamines in weight reduction programs altogether. However, for the man I mentioned above, diet pills were effective. He used them as a crutch for about six months and lost a lot of weight. That was quite a few years ago and he is still thin.

This fellow is the exception—not the rule. People usually deceive themselves while taking the pills into believing they are on their way to becoming thin. In reality, the pills can work against you because they don't require you to use any will power in resisting food. Your hunger symptoms are artificially masked. Once the effect wears off you often find yourself hungrier than ever and eat twice as much as you might have under ordinary circumstances.

I admit to having taken diet pills on occasion. And I'll tell you the truth: they don't work. Not only did I find myself overeating like crazy once the pill wore off, but when I considered my weight over a period of several months, I had accomplished absolutely zero. I was exactly the same weight as I had been, with or without the use of the pills.

Moreover, I found my heart racing, my memory disappearing and my mood becoming increasingly irritable.

No pills for me.

If you think there is a way around the prescription drug route by taking products sold over-the-counter, don't kid yourself. Anything that can be sold without a prescription won't be strong enough to effectively curb your appetite. If you read the ingredients labels you'll see that caffeine is frequently mentioned. If you know that caffeine acts as a temporary appetite depressant, you can save your money and simply brew a pot of coffee.

For those still not convinced that amphetamines are a "no-no" let me continue. Most of us are not on the mailing lists to receive the magazines our doctors read. In those which especially direct their attention to the bariatric (diet) physician you find pages of advertisements for various substances that promise to help patients depress their appetites.

One such ad was a beaut. I won't name the pharmaceutical company or the product. But it was for an amphetamine.

Nearly the entire ad is devoted to warnings, precautions, adverse reactions, and overdosage information. If you read that tolerance to the drug usually develops within a few weeks, you might still decide to use it for a short period. But if you knew that it is ill-advised to drive a car while taking it, or that you ought to be cautious even if you had only mild hypertension—or you might get palpitations, insomnia, even psychotic episodes (though a rare reaction) or diarrhea, etc., etc.—you might (I hope) decide against it.

The above information is included with the material doctors often remove from their prescription packages. If we had a chance to read it we'd probably swallow a lot less medication.

After I read that ad I became frightened. But forget fear. We all know that fear isn't the motivating factor in weight reduction. The fact is, as I said, these pills just don't work in the long run. I discovered that. I hope I have saved you the trouble of finding this out for yourself.

We must learn to recognize the signals our bodies give us telling us we are hungry. Once we do, we'll be better able to learn how to control ourselves. Eventually, we must develop improved eating habits. Pills will never develop anything but dependency.

Hunger pangs are a phenomenon some fat people never experience. People eat largely out of habit, in response to appetite, because they are bored, because they are upset or anxious or depressed or angry, etc. But rarely do heavy people eat because they are really hungry.

After I had lost a lot of weight, I found myself traveling a great deal on business trips. Danger! I was on a speaking tour and often did not have a chance to eat regular meals. Moreover, I was unfamiliar with some of the cities I visited and I was not carrying any "emergency" food with me. (You know what that is, right? It could be nonspoiling nutritious snack foods such as raisins, nuts, certain cheeses—but don't let it become candy bars! That defeats the purpose.)

For me, the carrying of emergency food began when I still believed I would starve to death if I didn't know when my next meal was coming. Later it became a realistic tool. If I have good snack foods handy when I'm traveling they will often help me overcome moments of hunger when I might otherwise go into uncontrolled eating.

One evening in a strange city, while waiting to be

interviewed I began to feel grouchy and tired. My host hadn't eaten dinner and suggested that I join him for a quick meal. The quick meal was a sandwich, the first one I'd eaten in years with two entire pieces of bread. Within a few minutes I felt revived. Afterwards I reflected that this may have been the first time in my adult life that I had experienced true hunger. I also had the opportunity to experience the direct effect of food as a source of energy.

I'm not suggesting that you wait as long as possible before eating. When you are extremely hungry it's difficult, if not impossible, to be selective about the food you eat. However, you might spend a few moments thinking about the last time you *really* allowed yourself to get hungry.

I have discovered that my energy level is especially high just before I find myself so hungry that I cannot think of anything except food. My body operates most efficiently when the food is just about all absorbed.

I'll illustrate this by giving you a reverse example. After a big lunch, it's hard to go back to work. It would be more natural to curl up into a little bundle and sleep. Countries where the siesta is practiced are those where the midday meal has traditionally been the largest. And, quite intelligently, in those countries, the people rest afterwards.

The feeling I'm talking about is opposite to this sleepy one. If lunchtime is at noon and you've had breakfast at 7:30 or 8:00 A.M., observe how you feel about 11:30 A.M. (provided you haven't eaten anything since your morning meal). It's an interesting exercise. Try it.

Now is a good time to discuss portions of food.

One of my favorite pastimes is reading restaurant reviews. Years ago a widely known food crtic described the portion size in one restaurant as "gross." Too much to eat! At that point in my life I couldn't imagine how anyone could give me too much to eat. On the contrary, if I read about such a restaurant I would immediately plan a visit. Then too, my favorite eating places were those that served buffet-style meals and encouraged you to go back as often as you liked. When they saw me coming they knew profits would be down that week.

Well, time has passed and now I understand about "gross" portions. The first moment I found myself saying "There's too much food here" I understood that food critic. As you read this you may not believe that there will be a time in your life when you have the same reaction. Believe me, it's true. I never thought it would happen to me and it did. And it can happen to you too.

I enjoy food more now than I ever did when it was quantity rather than quality that interested me. I also have discovered that recipes indicating that four pork chops serve four people aren't really crazy.

Americans eat too much. That's how we got fat in the first place. Our bodies need very little fuel (food) to keep running efficiently. I find that the less I eat (within reason, of course) the better I feel. I'm not suggesting that you starve yourself. But you should begin to think about how much food you are putting into your body.

I didn't get thin because I wanted to eat less and feel better. Not at all. But I did discover that I function well on small amounts of food; amounts so small that in the old days I would have doubted that they'd keep me alive.

When your next meal is in front of you, think about what you've just read. Look at your plate. Is all that food really for you? Or, should it be feeding your entire family? Be honest now. If you decide it's a proper portion for one, eat and enjoy it. But if you've begun to absorb some of what I've been saying, maybe, just maybe, you will push a teeny bit away. If you do, I know you are going to feel good about it later.

That leads me to a helpful reducing "trick." An acquaintance whom I hadn't seen for several months had lost a lot of weight. When I asked how he did it, he said he simply ate exactly half of whatever was put in front of him. Simple enough.

I tried this but I confess it was very difficult for me to leave food on my plate. Therefore, even as I give you this trick, I remind you that it may not be helpful for you. (Remember—not everything works for everybody.)

If you think you can handle this approach, try it. Results can be terrific and preparation is non-existent. Just eat half of everything on your plate. However, if you find yourself eating the icing half of a cocoanut cake, I think you're missing the point.

If you don't want to divide by two, just try eating less. In the January, 1980, issue of *Los Angeles* Magazine Dinah Shore says, "I eat less of everything. I don't want to feel deprived, so instead of a cup of mashed potatoes I have a teaspoonful."

Someone else I met invented his own way to control

what he eats. He designed a dinner plate with lots of small round spots on it. He doesn't take the first bite until all of the food has been fitted onto those small areas. By this time, he has lost much of his appetite. And he has insured that he will be eating small portions, since the food must fit on those spots.

It works for him.

A "trick" I've used was similar to that employed by a commercially sold diet item. The item is Ayds. Ayds is a nutritionally enriched caramel which is supposed to be eaten at specific times of the day to curb your appetite. A friend of mine tried Ayds. He loved them. His problem was that they tasted so good, he ate half the box of Ayds within a few minutes!

Ayds recently marketed an item called Ayds Droplets. They promise instant will power if you just put twelve "little drops in a drink before meals." And, they claim, a special "active ingredient" will help control even the most uncontrollable appetite. At the bottom of this ad, in very small type, is a warning that "Individuals with high blood pressure, heart disease, diabetes or thyroid disease should use only as directed by a physician."

I don't know about you, but when I read a warning like that I can't help but wonder what the "active ingredient" might be!

Well, my trick was sweet-tooth connected, like the old Ayds caramels. I would eat a piece of candy just before mealtimes. (I ignored my mother's voice, which nagged at my conscience about ruining my appetite. My goal was exactly that—to try to ruin my appetite.)

I found, for a while at least, the candy was very help-ful. I had to exercise a measure of control in order to limit myself to just one piece of candy, not the whole bagful. For insurance I carried precisely the amount of candy with me that would get me through the day. I guess that's why eating only half of what is on my plate doesn't work for me. I'd have to cut the portions in half *before* putting them on my plate for it to work for me!

The candy worked because I examined both my needs and my limitations. And that's what I'd like you to do. I'm not suggesting that you run out and fill your pockets with candy. Rather, think not only about *what* I did but *how* I did it.

As I said, eating half my food doesn't work for me. I guess as a child I was taught too well to clean my plate. Thus, if I had a pound of candy in my pocket I wouldn't be able to use this trick effectively either. So, I dis-ciplined myself by carrying only the amount of candy I needed. That way I also removed myself from the temptation of eating more.

Being on a diet is tough enough. You don't have to walk through fire to prove you can do it. Keep tempting foods away. I knew myself well enough to know that once I got hungry I would eat everything.

Candy may not be a good thing for you. Maybe it would trigger you to eat out of control. Maybe carrot sticks in a plastic bag will work. Or two pretzels before lunchtime. It's more important to pay attention to *how* I used the snack. Then you can apply the principle to some other food. Above all, you must learn to be completely honest with yourself about whether that item is going to help you, or whether you are merely looking for an excuse to eat.

You may believe you are honest with yourself. But remember when we discussed being honest about admitting you needed to lose weight? We all deceive ourselves from time to time. I delayed admitting I needed a diet until my husband told me in no uncertain terms that I was bursting at the seams.

Honesty with yourself is one of the most important ingredients for success in losing weight, and I will refer to it often. You must be able to look at yourself and understand and accept your strengths and your weaknesses. I'm not talking about how strong you *should* be; I'm talking about how strong you *are*. We are all temptable. Whoever denies this is not being honest.

Who ever said we have to be perfect? If you believe any human being is perfect, you still believe in the tooth fairy.

Successful weight loss does not come from being perfect. It is a result of understanding why you eat, and being realistic about how you are going to manage to keep yourself from eating things that make you fat— most of the time.

I have been telling you how I got thin and have stayed thin. And if you have been reading carefully, you will notice that I never tell you it's because I can control my food desires all the time. Rather, I am leveling with you about my stumbles and my successes.

Being honest with yourself is more important than

broadcasting your weight to your friends, spouse, or doctor. Sure, they can help, but in the final analysis they aren't carrying around the pounds. You are. And they aren't the ones pushing excess food into your mouth. You are. So, if you're serious not only about wanting to take off weight, but about keeping it off, this may be one of the most important concepts for you to digest.

Re-read the above paragraph and then put the book down for a few minutes and think about it.

Okay—now ask yourself this. Are you ready at this point in your life not only to take off weight, but to plan realistically about how you are going to eat in the future? Are you fed up with diets that don't seem to understand that you get hungry at 10:00 P.M. and not at 9:00 A.M.?

Are you ready to understand that it's going to take a lot of effort but that the rewards will be worth it? And do you really accept *full* responsibility for all the food you put into your body? Because no matter what the outside pressures or temptations, the truth is that *you* respond to those pressures and temptations by eating. You shovel food into your mouth. There are other ways to respond.

As soon as you accept total responsibility for your own actions, you can make conscious decisions about altering them.

Remember, this is the turning point—the time of your life when you are about to change *forever* from an overweight person into one who can be thin. I'm not going to do it for you. Your doctor isn't going to do it for you. Nobody but you can do it for you. *And you can do it!*

I did!

Now set the book down and review this chapter in your mind.

NINE COMMANDMENTS
FOR WEIGHT CONTROL

1. Think of yourself as a thin person

2. Plan your meals and snacks: know ahead of time exactly what you will eat and how much

3. For the first week, avoid all restaurants

4. Do not read or watch television while you eat: concentrate on your food

5. Never eat anything while standing up

6. Put your fork or spoon down after each mouthful. Don't refill it until you've swallowed

7. Chew slowly. Taste what you are eating

8. Fill your plate only with the amount of food you want. Do not eat from platters on the table. No seconds.

9. Always leave some food on your plate

More Help

Y ou and I are doing magic together.

Are some of the tricks I've shared with you tricks you already knew? Was there at least one that is new to you? Good. Then I'm helping. I don't expect you to come to this book a "virgin." But do come to it with an open mind.

I repeat, one approach will seem tailored for one individual's success, while another person might find the same technique utterly frustrating and self-defeating.

Let's look at an example. Some years ago a reducing aid called Metrecal was put on the market. For those of you with short memories, Metrecal was a concoction of vitamins, minerals and a measured quantity of calories. In the beginning it came as a powder and you had to add water and mix your own liquid nourishment.

Metrecal had the advantage of being a complete meal in a glass for those who didn't want to bother putting together their own menu of nutritious and weight-watching foods. It came in a variety of delicious-sounding flavors like strawberry, Dutch chocolate, and coffee. Metrecal was followed by many similar controlled calorie preparations.

A woman I knew really got into Metrecal. She learned to love its flavors. She used it faithfully. The only problem was she wasn't losing weight. When queried as to how she used Metrecal which, after all, contained a controlled number of calories, she insisted that in the morning, every morning, all she would drink was Metrecal. When pressed, she reluctantly added one additional item of information. With the Metrecal, she ate a large piece of danish pastry.

Examine the "diet" foods that you are eating if they don't seem to be helping. Could it be that you are supplementing too?

My friend Bill Gaines of *Mad* magazine also used Metrecal, but he did it a bit more effectively. By the time he became interested in Metrecal it was available in premixed, measured portions in cans.

He too loved the flavors. His trick was to put the cans into the freezer. When he was ready to have his Metrecal he opened the top of the can and spooned it out, pretending it was ice cream. You can be sure it took a lot of time and effort to dig out the contents. Thus, the Metrecal portion went quite a distance, and satisfied his need for "dessert."

Speaking of foods that are labeled "diet"—are they really worth it? I used to buy diet cookies and diet candies. The amusing thing I discovered is that they often aren't much lower in calories than nondiet items. Read the caloric content of some of these so-called diet items and you too may be surprised to learn that a plain

cookie has fewer calories than the one you have purchased as a substitute. And be assured, you'll pay a lot
more for the diet cookie.

Even the Weight Watchers prepared frozen dinners
sometimes contain more calories than a meal you can
put together yourself.

I reached a point when I decided that if I felt eating
cookies was putting pounds on, I shouldn't be looking
for a low-calorie substitute. I should be looking for a way
to live without them, at least until I felt I had learned
how to introduce cookies into my life without consuming
more than I planned to eat. Then I would eat cookies
and enjoy them. And everyone knows that nondiet
cookies beat the taste of the sugarless kind any day
in the week.

As for Bill Gaines, who liked to think of his Metrecal
as ice cream—he readily admitted Metrecal didn't compare to the real thing.

One more suggestion if desserts are your passion: eat
yours as your first course. That way you'll really enjoy
it and probably not eat more than your portion. You
might even save a taste for last, and so start and end
your meal with dessert!

Exercise is frequently suggested as a method to reduce.
If you already play tennis three times a week, chances
are you probably are also reasonably trim. However, if
you are a weekend jock, exercise might be helpful, if
for no other reason than part of the time you might
otherwise spend eating you are now spending in physical
pursuits.

Don't begin a vigorous jogging program, however, believing that the exercise alone will be enough to take off the unwanted pounds. Exercise *can* help keep your body firm and change your contours, but it's not realistic to believe that even if you exercise like mad you can get thin by burning up the calories you consume when overeating.

Here's an idea of the amount of exercise you might expect to do in order to burn up some calories:

An english muffin contains 180 calories. Eat one if you choose. To write it off you could jump into a pool and swim vigorously for 21 minutes.

Have that jelly donut. Afterwards, work off the 226 calories by walking for 43 minutes, or by running 13.

Or, why not spoon two tablespoons of sour cream into your baked potato? That will cost 57 calories which you can bicycle away in 9 minutes.

If you've always wondered how many calories are expended in an hour of scrubbing floors, it's between 200 and 250 (it depends, of course, on how vigorously you work) but sweeping floors will use up only between 75 and 125 calories for the hour's work.

Keep in mind that one pound of body fat contains the equivalent of 3500 calorie units of energy. It's not hard to figure out, therefore, why you can't count exercise alone to get you thin.

Our bodies are not simple machines. You can't merely exchange a certain amount of exercise for caloric intake and expect to balance things out. It just doesn't work that neatly. Besides, are you aware of how long and how exhausting twenty-one minutes of vigorous swimming actually is? Try it.

I'm not an athlete, but a few years ago I decided I would jog a mile every day. After many months I finally worked up to the mile. I was no Roger Bannister or even a Glenn Cunningham. I did my mile in about ten minutes. For me this was quite an accomplishment. However, I never saw any weight reduction that I could attribute to the running.

Many people worry that exercise will increase their appetite. I find (and many others with whom I've spoken agree) the opposite is true. I recently took up horseback riding. It involves a great deal more exertion than I had anticipated. I enjoy it more than any exercise I've ever done. I am so exhilarated at the end of a riding lesson that I literally have no appetite. It's as if the challenge and excitement have filled me up. Frequently, I use that feeling after the lesson to skip a meal.

After analyzing this reaction I came to the conclusion that part of the fulfillment is from being totally involved. Ironically, there just are too few times when we food-oriented people find ourselves in that position.

So much in our daily lives revolves around food. We meet for dinner, discuss business at lunch, socialize over cocktails. It's downright antisocial to suggest to friends that we simply want to meet and share their company, without involving food or drink.

Try to change the focus in your life away from food. It would be easier to resist eating unnecessary calories if they weren't there in the first place.

As for becoming totally involved, if you think about

the way you spend your time, you'll find too few moments when you are so immersed in doing something that you aren't planning your next snack break.

Wouldn't it be interesting to consider those moments when you *are* so occupied. Then you can start planning to increase the time you spend productively in nonfood pursuits so you can increase their frequency.

When Lyle Stuart was on his protein-sparing fast he was amazed by how much free time he had since he wasn't spending any time eating. I'm not suggesting you give up eating, but try to think of things you enjoy doing and try to do more of them. You may find you spend less time eating, too.

If exercise is something you enjoy, get more involved in it. But, go easy. If you ordinarily do little more than lift yourself from your chair to change the station on the television tube (and alas, most new sets don't even require that: you lie there like a lump and push buttons) get a medical checkup before you begin jogging several miles a day.

Before you begin *any* strenuous exercise program you must make sure your body can handle it. Certainly, if you are carrying around a great deal of excess weight you especially want to make certain any change in your physical activity won't overtax your body.

If you want to exercise but believe you can't find the time, or place, try jogging in place in front of the television set. Or, do ten jumping jacks while you're waiting for the elevator to reach your floor. (Make sure you're alone!) Try dancing around the house. All of these activities not only get your body moving, but act as antidepressants. They are good methods of letting out emotions that are bottled up within us.

There *is* one form of exercise everyone can do. And before belittling the benefits, remember, it is better than nothing at all and requires little or no preparation. And don't forget, it's time spent away from food!

The exercise I refer to is walking.

You'd be surprised at how few people there are who walk. Or maybe you wouldn't be surprised. Begin by walking a few minutes each day—perhaps instead of driving to one destination. A side benefit of walking is that you will find yourself examining your surroundings more carefully than you probably have in years.

If you really get into it, you might find yourself working up to walking an energetic mile daily. (That's only four times around a quarter-mile high school track.) Even if you don't change your food consumption, it could result in dropping 10 pounds in a year.

"Roving" (actually brisk walking) is recommended by Nathan Pritikin, widely known for his best-selling book, *The Pritikin Program,* co-authored with Patrick M. McGrady, Jr.

An earlier work, *Live Longer Now: The First One Hundred Years of Your Life,* discussed the benefits of a program offered by Pritikin at his Longevity Center in Santa Barbara, California. The program focuses on patients with serious degenerative diseases such as hypertension, angina, atherosclerosis, arthritis and diabetes.

As reported by Andrew Kopkind in an article published in *Politics Today* magazine (March/April, 1978), the patient enters the center for a "costly 26-day treatment program. . . . The program includes 'roving' (brisk walking) and a very spartan diet . . ."

Probably Pritikin's most outstanding success is Eula Weaver, a woman over eighty who entered with a history of incapacitating heart problems. After a year of diet and exercise "she tossed out eight medicines she had been taking. After two years she was jogging and riding a stationary bicycle." She eventually won gold medals in mile and half-mile events in the Senior Olympics held each year in Irvine, California.

Are you about to tell me that the above description has exhausted you to the extent that you will hang up your jogging shoes forever?

Do you completely reject the idea of regular exercise? Don't leave me! I'm flexible. I have other suggestions.

One important point: you must employ an aid in order for it to help, because just thinking about it is not the same as doing it!

You might try cooking. Cooking? Wouldn't that put you in the very path of temptation? Odd as it seems, some people find that they can spend hours preparing elaborate meals for their family and never eat a bite. I too have discovered that occasionally the preparation of food "fills" me up. Whether it's the aroma of food cooking or, again, the involvement in the activity as an art, by the time the food is on the table I often feel like I've already eaten.

You might observe too that many professional cooks, cookbook writers, and food critics are quite thin. They have learned how to live with food as their life's work and not get fat.

On the other hand, there is the woman who was so much of an unconscious nibbler that she found it necessary to wear a surgical mask in the kitchen so she could not feed herself. Even so, from time to time she would find herself trying to pass bits of food through the gauze!

So, before you embrace this as a good idea, consider whether you are unconsciously seeking another excuse to get close to food.

If cooking turns on your appetite, obviously this is not for you. In which case, remove yourself completely from food preparation. True, if you are responsible for preparing the meals for your family this isn't always easy to accomplish. However, if you have youngsters who are old enough to help out in the kitchen, this might be the perfect time for them to learn how to cook. You can turn their lessons into benefits for you. All the mistakes they make while learning may bring food to the table that is easy to resist. And that means less going into your body.

For those of you who live alone, here's another suggestion. Train yourself to shop only for the exact amounts and kinds of food you are going to consume. Take a list with you. Buy *nothing* that isn't on your list. This will cut down on the impulse shopping you do. Forget about bargains for a while. Many such bargains are on large or economy sized items. You may be saving some pennies but you will be spending them on unwanted calories.

Learning how to shop while trying to reduce is very important. If you always keep in mind that supermarkets are designed to lure you into impulsive food acquisitions that you hadn't planned to make, you'll find it easier to resist. It's you against them. The supermarket is enemy territory!

In *Lose Weight Naturally: Prevention Magazine's No-Diet No-Willpower Method,* Mark Bricklin offers helpful ideas for shopping. He cites the fact that 78 percent of shoppers never planned to buy any snack foods when they entered the supermarkets. Notice, when you are in the store, how most candy is placed at a five-year-old child's eye level. This is not pure accident. Notice how easily they can reach out and grab and then beg you to buy the item!

When you're at the checkout counter you frequently find yourself waiting on long lines facing a tempting candy bar display. This goes for "health food" stores too. The fact that a candy bar is made with honey or brown sugar doesn't help the dieter.

Okay, so how can you fight it? I've already told you to prepare a shopping list before entering the store. You've got to be to develop plan equal to the von Clausewitz strategy of war.

Bricklin suggests that if you insist on bringing home snack foods, at least decide *before* you enter the store just what they are going to be.

Why let yourself be tempted by seductive packages? If you *must* have snack foods, limit yourself to those you can eat without going crazy. If you can't resist eating an entire bag of peanuts, don't buy one in the first place.

Of course, there is another point of view about snacking. If you decide that you would rather forgo tickets to the next Super Bowl than give up your between-meal snacks, you could find things that are nutritious and not total calorie wasters. This will take a little effort.

The United States Agriculture Department offers you a series of glossy, full-color magazines entitled *Food*. In these you will find suggestions and recipes for snacks ranging from pickled eggs (only 80 calories each) to beef tacos (270 calories).

I'd go easy on the beef tacos, though, because to my thinking 270 calories starts sounding more like a meal than a snack.

However, if you must snack, you'd be better off eating marinated vegetables (about 75 calories per cup) than hand-dipped chocolates.

If you want more information about nutritious snacks, write to the Consumer Information Center, Department 693-G, Pueblo, Colorado 81009.

Not all dieters will have the patience to prepare snacks from elaborate recipes. All too often we find ourselves wanting a snack "right now" and few will head to the kitchen to start cooking.

Whether you are cooking your snack foods or shopping for them, be sure you make conscious decisions.

One other suggestion about going to the market. Never shop for food when you've just been shopping for other items. You will be tired and might be tempted to "reward" yourself with food because you have been on your feet all day.

Don't keep food around "just in case" someone drops in. If your friends visit you only for the cake and cookies you serve, let them adjust to your new lifestyle. Genuine friends will be supportive of your efforts. And it will give you a chance to begin changing the focus of your socializing from food to people.

Tell your friends they can count on you only for coffee, tea or low calorie beverages. If they need to nibble let them bring along the things they want to eat. And then make sure they take the leftovers home when they leave.

Another word about goodies. (Or should we refer to them as "baddies"?) People who have young children often use the kids as an excuse to stock supplies of Oreo cookies, chocolate bars, caramel popcorn and such junk foods in the pantry. As I discovered from doing this myself, my daughter, Jenny, not only doesn't need the Lorna Doones and Hershey Kisses, she actually prefers fresh fruit. I was the one chomping down most of the empty calories, not Jenny and her friends.

It's interesting to observe Jenny growing up without a house filled with empty calories. She doesn't miss them because most of the time they aren't there. Further, her school has requested that parents not send the kids to school with lunch boxes filled with such items.

Jenny's is not the only school finally getting wise to the need to provide children with better lunches than have been served in past years. Many communities are making strides towards dumping the empty calorie foods from school cafeterias and bringing in nutritious items.

Dieting Is Hard Work

You and I know that dieting is hard work. The very idea of beginning a new reducing program is enough to depress some people and set them off on an eating spree. But this isn't a new diet; it's the beginning of a new life.

Taking responsibility for your life can be quite a turn on. Finding methods for getting thin will give you a rich sense of accomplishment.

This time you *can* win the war against fat—and not just the battle to take it off. I told you before: This *is* war. Think of your diet aids and controls as weapons in the struggle. Change your weapons from time to time if it will keep you from becoming bored. *Boredom is a danger signal for dieters.* It ranks with anxiety as one of the two most dangerous anti-food-control bombs.

Just as not every reducing idea will appeal to everyone, variation of those concepts that *do* help is also a good idea. I change my "weapons" often. Something that might have been a terrific idea last week may not help me to battle the temptation of those potato chips tonight.

The deep satisfaction that success brings can carry you through stressful periods of your life, and no longer will you misuse those moments to succumb to self-destructive food gorging.

Most of us know all too well how anxiety frequently leads to overeating. It probably accounts for hundreds of added pounds. (Singer Jan Bart once wrote a book titled "I Lost a Thousand Pounds.")

Perhaps you'll be inspired by the story of a woman I know who handled stress and weight control in a special, productive way.

This woman had gone through a year of constant changes in her life. These were both emotional and physical. In fact, in the period of one year she became deeply involved with a man and moved across the country to Oregon to be with him. By the end of the year the relationship had ended and she moved back to New York. During this time her career underwent several changes, and as her income level changed, she moved from one apartment to another.

I did not mention in the beginning of this story that the woman was overweight. Of course, you knew that. However, during this period she had been losing weight —more weight than she had ever been able to lose in her life.

When people are under the kind of stress I've just described *and* they are also trying to reduce, few have the determination to keep going. Ironically, when I asked the woman how she had handled her weight during this time, she told me that she had not only managed to keep from gaining, she had even reduced further.

She explained: "Since I had very little control over what was going on in my life, I realized the one thing I *could* control was what was going into my body."

Dieting gave her a sense of control and success.

This story can be an inspiration if you're a person who looks for every excuse to get off your diet.

Lots of us like to look at famous people as inspirational figures to model ourselves after.

From time to time we read how a movie star keeps his or her figure. I'm fascinated by these articles. It's always interesting to learn new methods. But there's also a certain satisfaction in discovering that even the rich and famous have weight problems.

Angie Dickinson made a strong impression. She said that one trick she uses to curb her appetite is to brush her teeth frequently. Now maybe it's only a publicity story, but I tried it and it helped. You might try it too. Naturally, we don't want to whip out our brushes at the dinner table or in a fancy restaurant. But this might be the secret you've been waiting for all your life.

Let's try, however, to keep our methods somewhat sensible, not like that of the woman who once confided that her secret was never to swallow anything. She carried a Styrofoam cup with her and after chewing her food thoroughly, she spit it into the cup. I suspect she "ate" most of her meals alone.

There are enough ways to cut down on eating without resorting to antisocial behavior. Your goal is to learn how to live with food and be in control of what you eat, not to eliminate food from your life entirely.

Another widespread unconscious habit among dieters is to forget some of what we have eaten.

Early in our marriage, my husband tried to reduce. I occasionally asked him what he had eaten that day. He dutifully recited it all. But it wasn't all. Too often he conveniently "forgot" the apple pie and coffee he had in midafternoon.

Here's one way to make yourself more acutely aware of your habits:

Write down what you eat and when you eat it. Don't try to change your eating patterns. What you're trying to accomplish initially is to become conscious of your eating patterns. The relearning will come soon enough. Carry a notebook with you and each time you put *any-thing* in your mouth, write it down. Even if it's only a stick of sugarless gum or a peanut.

Don't skip anything!

Be sure to record the time you eat. I'm aware that this exercise, if carried on too long, could become a pain, so let's limit the timespan. But do it for at least two days.

Then look at your records. If you have kept them faithfully you should begin to see a pattern. As an example, here is the record of a friend who took my suggestion and did exactly this:

DAY ONE:

8:00 A.M.	½ cup orange juice
NOON	chicken thigh and leg in a tomato and eggplant sauce (approx. ½–¾ cup of sauce)
3:00 P.M.	1 cup frozen vanilla yogurt (maybe more)
6:30 P.M.	2 vodka gimlets
	Undetermined amount of Fritos
7:30 P.M.	Chinese/wok style chicken with zucchini in a hoison sauce 1½–2½ cups
	salad: Boston lettuce, ½ tomato, cucumber, scallion, bottled dressing
	½ bottle dry white wine.
9:15 P.M.	¼ slice cantaloupe
10:00 P.M.	⅔ pint vanilla ice cream

DAY TWO:

8:15 A.M.	1 cup orange juice
	1 cup coffee
4:00 P.M.	undetermined (but not that much since I polished off most of the bag the day before) of Fritos
	2 cans of beer
8:00 P.M.	three pieces of cheese and mushroom and pepperoni pizza
	club soda

DAY THREE:

	(a terrible food hangover)
7:45 A.M.	1 cup coffee
12:30 P.M.	small salad—iceberg lettuce, ½ tomato, 1 tbs. bermuda onion, bottled dressing
5:30 P.M.	1 scotch sour (made with lo-cal sour mix and a spritz of lemon juice to make it palatable)
	a few nibbles of Fritos
9:15 P.M.	approx. two cups of wok style shrimp dish—tomato paste, scallions, ginger, some brown sugar, soy sauce
	½ bottle dry white wine

DAY FOUR:

8:30 A.M.	1 soft-boiled egg
	¼ cup of orange juice
	1 cup coffee, black
NOON	1 small slice of ham
	1 cup coffee
5:30 P.M.	1 bourbon sour (not made with lo-cal sour mix)
7:00 P.M.	salad—iceberg lettuce, 1 large mushroom, some tomatoes, oil and vinegar dressing
	chicken in white sauce with artichoke hearts
	1 stalk broccoli
	3 glasses dry white wine
8:00 P.M.	Several more cups of coffee

Now keep in mind that the purpose of reproducing a real food record is to make you aware of food. Let's analyze my friend's record and see what we learn.

First, this is a person who enjoys food. Enjoys it enough to cook and vary the menu a great deal. It is also the record of someone who enjoys wine and cocktails. But not especially desserts. My friend eats balanced meals but occasionally nibbles more than desired.

There's a lot that can be modified. (Don't forget this list does not reflect weight-conscious eating. It's simply a record of everything eaten, without thinking about dieting.)

Now the time comes to ask yourself, if this was *your* food chart, what would you suggest if you wanted to design a reducing plan keeping in mind your food desires and your weight goal?

My recommendations? For one thing, I would simplify the recipes. The more ingredients added to a dish, the more difficult to keep track of the calories. At restaurants I tend to avoid foods when I don't know what goes into their preparation. (At home you can keep track, but nevertheless, elaborate combinations can easily add up to more calories than you might really want to eat.)

Next, I would suggest that my friend cut down on alcohol. Not only does alcohol add huge numbers of calories, but it can stimulate the appetite so that you lose control over eating. (It could be the reason the Fritos were eaten.)

Note that I didn't suggest cutting out the booze altogether. Chances are that would produce a feeling of deprivation which might drive one further into eating. Just cut down.

Becoming aware of what you eat is a giant step in changing your eating behavior. Only when you are aware can you modify. If you never become aware, you'll continue the same patterns that caused the problem.

SEVEN STEPS TO GAIN CONTROL OF WHAT YOU EAT

1. For two consecutive days, write down everything you put into your mouth. Estimate the quantities. Record the time.

2. At the end of the two days, put a check mark next to those foods which were pure snack or junk food.

3. Circle all bread, crackers, cakes, candy, ice cream and other desserts.

4. Ask yourself if you truly enjoyed every one of the checked and/or circled foods.

5. Rewrite the list, cutting out at least two things that you circled or checked on your list.

6. Ask yourself if your new list won't give you as much satisfaction as the list of foods you actually consumed.

7. Prepare a menu for the next twenty-four hours and stick to it.

Conscious
and Unconscious Eating

I can't overemphasize the importance of becoming aware of the food you eat. Let me tell you about a friend who thought he knew what he ate, but really didn't.

During the day and even through dinner Dan Gardner ate moderately. He couldn't understand why he had such a decidedly large paunch where there previously had been a flat stomach. He thought about the foods he ate each day and his eating was certainly within reasonable limits. He was truly perplexed.

He discussed the problem with his wife, Joan, and she agreed to try to help him by observing his habits.

It didn't take long for Dan's wife to solve the mystery. Each morning, a great deal of food was missing from the refrigerator. She had noticed this before, but since Dan and his wife had two teen-agers, she assumed that it was the pair of "growing children" who were snacking after dinner.

129

Dan's wife questioned the children. They assured her they weren't eating the food. And so she confronted Dan with the obvious solution: he had eaten the food himself.

Dan thought about it. He was a modest eater at meals. But late at night, usually after Joan had fallen asleep, he would get out of bed and wander into the kitchen for a "light bite."

The fact is that somehow, in Dan's perception, the food he ate at night "didn't really count."

Dan is with the book advertising department of *The New York Times*. He deals with complaints, crises, deadlines and a bucketful of anxieties all day long. And he handles them well. But somehow they gang up on him when he is lying in bed.

Joan decided to convince herself. One night she pretended to be sleeping. A half hour later, Dan arose. He seemed to be sleepwalking.

Joan followed Dan down the stairs. She waited until the refrigerator door opened and closed. Again and again. Then she walked in to a startled husband. He was into a Dagwood sandwich—a hero roll piled high with a little bit of everything!

Dan expressed such innocent surprise that Joan knew she had a real problem. Like a stubborn alcoholic, Dan couldn't relate his growing paunch to "these little occasional late night snacks."

It took a week of soul-searching for Joan and the children to come up with a possible solution to keep Dan from becoming a baby elephant.

They decided to secure the refrigerator.

They hired a locksmith who gave them a chain and a hefty lock. Each night after dinner, Joan would chain the refrigerator door and lock the lock.

It worked!

Very quickly Dan Gardner began to shed weight. The paunch became smaller. It seemed as if a happy ending was in view.

And then, without reason, Dan began to balloon up again. And in the mornings, when Joan undid the lock and chain, there was food missing from the refrigerator shelves.

The family was faced with a new mystery.

This one was solved with logic.

Dan was no Houdini. He obviously had discovered where the key was hidden.

Again Joan did the "make believe you're sleeping" number. Sure enough, twenty minutes later Dan was on his way.

The key had been hidden under a can of Bon Ami scouring powder in a closet.

What to do? Joan confided the problem to a friend. The friend made a suggestion.

The next night when Dan reached under the Bon Ami can, instead of a key, he found a note. It read: "Not tonight, Danny Boy! The phantom strikes again!"

It was signed by the friend who'd made the suggestion. Dan was so frustrated, upset and angry that he confessed that he was tempted to make a 2 A.M. telephone call to the friend to tell him off!

It's an amusing story but I must point out that what Joan did in locking the food away was a short-term, not a long-term solution. Nobody can do it for you. *You have to want to do it yourself.*

Are people often unconscious of their eating? More often than you might imagine. I think of the case of John MacArthur, who was one of America's authentic billionaires.

MacArthur could have bought almost anything he saw. His vast holdings exceeded those possessed by kings of old. And yet, deep down, he was still the insecure little boy who had run away from home.

One symptom emerged when he attended a party. MacArthur would literally stuff his pockets with the (free) sandwiches.

If he saw the half full punch bowl on leaving the party, he couldn't resist picking it up with both hands and pouring the contents into his mouth.

John MacArthur, billionaire, could never understand why he had that protruding paunch that gave him his pear shape!

Does the body know when it is too fat? Research at the University of Washington Medical School in Seattle indicates that in non-fat people, the level of insulin in the cerebrospinal fluid gives the body a signal.

The researchers found that they could cause baboons to eat less and lose weight by injecting insulin directly into their brains.

The general belief is that fat people produce insulin in normal amounts but that the brain's insulin-detecting mechanism may be faulty. Thus, obese people need higher levels of insulin to signal their bodies to "Okay. Stop eating now!"

But alas, medical scientists haven't yet figured out how to raise the levels of insulin in the brain without causing problems in other parts of the body.

Oh well, so much for another simple-seeming solution!

Cravings: Making Them Work for You

Two chapters ago, we analyzed the food records of my friend and learned a lot about that person's likes and food involvement. You made your own record and you examined it in pretty much the same way.

What can you do to alter your food habits? Awareness is a big step. But what about those things you just can't live without? If they are taken away, it will be the end of the world. Or at least it feels that way right now.

We all have cravings. In order to learn how to deal with these you must do some serious analysis of your food needs.

First of all, in the words of psychologist Dr. Albert Ellis, "You don't need what you want."

Read that again.

It's a deceptively simple statement. But it can apply to many things in your life. We may *want* many things, but how many of them are necessities?

If you learn to understand this concept you will have moved further toward conquering overeating.

Food is an emotional issue. Some people aren't necessarily on diets, but they have neurotic food attitudes. My former father-in-law had a large family, and an adequate income. When the family met for a reunion and he knew he was going to take everyone to a restaurant for dinner, he always ate at home first. Somehow he felt he was saving the money his meal would cost!

Money isn't an issue with the greedy eater. Here, it's the belief, imagined or otherwise, that this is the last chance he or she is ever going to have to eat the kinds of food that are in front of them! (As if cheesecake will never make another appearance!)

You recognize how silly this is. But you've got to learn to believe that you can go out and buy that particular food or something just as good anytime you want to.

If you have between-meal hunger and simply cannot control it, trying to attain that control may be counter-productive—at least at this time in your life. Don't forget, we want to get you going in a positive direction. That means dealing with *your* reality, not the reality of some "ideal." So, if you decide you want to eat between meals, perhaps it would be wise to think in terms of a longer period of time to lose weight. Or, as I suggested earlier, how about trying to find out how to make those snacks nutritious?

But what if you don't care about nutrition? What if the only "snack" that will do the trick is a Big Mac or an ice cream soda?

Have you thought about the ice cream soda? Are you

making a conscious decision that you want it? Are you being impulsive? Who is in the driver's seat, you or the food?

If I asked myself all these questions and could honestly answer that *I* had made the decision to have it, I would have the best ice cream soda I could buy. I would enjoy it thoroughly.

Get guilt out of your life! But be aware that you *will* have to pay for your snack by putting your weight goal back somewhat. However, if the snack is important enough, maybe it's worth the price.

You decide.

Let me give you an analogy, using a non-weight situation. A woman I knew announced to her husband that she wanted to go back to college and get her bachelor's degree. She was fifty years old at the time. Her husband said she was being silly.

"After all," he pointed out, "you'll be fifty-four years old by the time you finish."

"Well," she responded, "I'm going to be fifty-four in four more years anyway, so I may as well be fifty-four *with* my degree!"

You may feel that by extending your weight-loss program you will be wasting time. But don't forget, like the above woman, time is going to pass anyway, so if you get thin a bit slower, you'll still be using the time positively.

If you tailor your reducing plan to your own lifestyle you will be successful. You will also enjoy taking control of your life. Fit that between-meal hunger into your plan and make it work for you.

You can still have snacks and make them work for you. Let me repeat this. It is very important. Each time you decide you are going to eat something between meals promise yourself that you are going to think about it. By that I mean, ask yourself, "Do I really want this?" If the answer is yes, have it. But if you are making excuses to overeat, don't have it. Pass up the snack. Make sure *you* are deciding, not the food.

Don't ever forget that *you* are the one who decided that your goal will take a longer time to reach because *you* have *chosen* to eat that snack.

At some point you may decide to alter your decision. Or, perhaps not. Just keep yourself aware. And eliminate unconscious eating.

Let's go back to cravings. I understand these very well. We all have them. You don't have to be in the advanced stages of pregnancy to understand strong food desires.

I once heard about a school teacher who had a weight problem. She was at her desk when the class returned from lunch break. One of the students walked in nibbling on a donut.

After taking a few bites the students tossed it into the wastepaper basket. From the moment the remains of that donut hit the basket the teacher could think of nothing else. When the bell rang and the class filed out at the end of the day, she dove for the donut.

Sad? Funny? A bit of both. But which of us can't identify with that story, if only in a small way?

Perhaps if the teacher had understood and accepted

her cravings and fit them into her food program she wouldn't have gone for the donut.

Why you crave certain food is complicated. It all depends on what food means to you. Is it the comfort it promises but never seems to deliver because once you eat you suffer from guilt? Are you driven by anxiety?

For whatever reason we desire foods, it is obvious that heavy people, or even people who have their weight under control—but are food-oriented—live different lives than those for whom food is merely a daily routine.

Have you ever watched thin people eat? It's fascinating because it's so different from the way food-oriented people eat. For instance, a young attorney I know, for whom food is merely a means of nourishment, told me that sometimes he gets so busy at work he forgets to eat lunch.

Forgets to eat lunch!

I have been in situations where there are heated discussions going on and all I can think about is when and what I'm going to eat. Ah well, I can never be that attorney, but at least I've learned to understand and cope with my food desires.

I'm not here to analyze you but to help you do that for yourself. You do crave certain foods and if you believe you can't live without satisfying that need, you probably will be better off accepting your need rather than constantly battling against it. That way you will diffuse the explosive potential of denying the need.

I'm here to help you handle your food needs realistically. If you crave certain foods, include them in your life. Otherwise you'll soon feel deprived.

If boredom is one of the reasons people overeat, deprivation is the major cause of diet failure.

Everytime you start a new diet, you feel a sense of
doom, right? Isn't it because you begin with the belief
that you are putting behind you all the foods you love—
forever?

What I'm telling you is quite different.

You don't have to live the rest of your life without
mashed potatoes. Or French fries. Or chocolate pudding. Or whatever it is you love.

I'm telling you that if you want to lose weight, and
keep it off, you *must* include those favorite foods in
your life. Otherwise you will feel deprived, and feelings
of deprivation lead to feeling sorry for yourself.

The next step is rationalizing, and then comes the
binge.

The most effective way to short circuit a binge is to
plan to have the goody you crave. But—when you control your food you also control the manner in which you
will eat that special item. I'll show you how to make
your cravings work for rather than against you.

Is this childish?

Not at all. In fact, it's being more adult than you've
been in a long time. None of us is perfect. (If you were
perfect you wouldn't be reading this book.)

My craving is for the perfect chocolate chip cookie.
I like sweets. I know I probably would be a few pounds
lighter without them, but I have thought about how important sweets are to me and have decided that for me,
they're worth having. And so I include them in my eat-

ing program. I have made the decision. Nobody ever got fat from eating one chocolate chip cookie, or even one ice cream soda!

Here's how to make this work for you. First decide whether you want to include in your diet some item that you feel is worth having. Plan pecisely when you will eat it and limit yourself to that single food.

Promise yourself that you will wait for the moment you set aside and keep your word to yourself. When you do this you won't nibble on lots of other things because you can wait for the time set aside for this pleasure. And it is genuinely pleasurable.

Infants demand instant gratification. When their bellies are empty, they cry out for food. But you're no longer an infant and get much more gratification out of planning and shaping when and where you'll indulge yourself. That, after all, is one thing that separates us from infants.

Somtimes, I'll admit, my concentration is intense about that goody. At other times I find that I have out-witted myself. When the hour rolls around for the promised chocolate chip cookie, I find I'm too full from having eaten dinner or too sleepy, and then, I skip it.

What is *your* favorite treat? French bread, chopped liver, caviar? Have it—but *you* make the decision.

INTERMISSION EXERCISE

Examine your food cravings.

Do you have any? Is there one very special food you have denied yourself because you feel it is a "no-no"?

Select that food and once, just once plan to have it.

Plan exactly where you will sit, and the time you will choose to eat it. At that moment, go ahead, and fully enjoy it. See if it doesn't satisfy you. And see, too, if it hasn't put off a potential eating binge.

Have You Heard
This One Before?

I could have called this chapter "A Review of All the Diets of the Twentieth Century," but I like this title better. The fact is, there is very little new under the sun in dieting. Whether they call it Stillman, Atkins, Pritikin, or Scarsdale, most of what they have to say has been said before.

If you think I exaggerate, let's examine the program Dr. Atkins calls "The Diet Revolution."

When Dr. Robert Atkins burst onto the scene a few years ago with his "revolutionary" diet, he proposed high-fat, high-protein foods. The main appeal was in that magical word, "unlimited." Dr. Atkins promised that you could eat as much as you wanted of his "unlimited" foods and you would lose weight.

Your body would deliberately be put into a state of ketosis. Ketosis occurs when triglycerides (stored fat in the body) are broken down. This condition produces free fatty acids and glycerol.

143

Some of the free fatty acids go right to the lean body mass for fuel; the rest is partially oxidized (burned up) by the liver into "ketone bodies."

The debate continues as to whether ketosis is a harmful state for the body to be in. According to Dr. Atkins, it's wonderful. As a matter of fact he claims ketosis is a sign "that unwanted fat is being burned up as fuel."

But . . . if you are a diabetic, beware, for ketosis could develop into acidosis. And if you're pregnant, ketosis could seriously threaten the fetus.

My philosophy is, anything that can harm an unborn child may be able to harm me too. However, lots of people welcomed not having to count calories. You could indulge your desire for high-fat foods which tend to make you feel full longer.

Watch out for any diet that promises that you can eat as much as you want.

That's a misleading statement since as much as *you* want may be much more, or less, than I want. For instance, my good friend Bill Gaines, publisher of *Mad* magazine, thought he'd try Atkins' program. Bill loves butter, steak and heavy cream. It seemed tailor-made for him.

Telling Bill that he could eat "as much as you want" didn't take into consideration his very large capacity. He became a patient of Dr. Atkins. He gained weight.

Thus. Dr. Atkins' Revolution doesn't work for everyone. Like many one-sided diets, this one really ends up working because you simply eat fewer calories. No matter how much you may like steak, the premise is that eventually you will grow tired, yes, even of steak, and cut down on your portions.

One of the more serious criticisms of this diet is that it is high in saturated fat and cholesterol. If your blood cholesterol level is high, better stay away. The danger of increasing your cholesterol is not the only worry to concern yourself about while eating a high fat diet. Such a regime may also result in kidney and/or heart disease, vomiting or excessive uric acid in the blood which can lead to gout.

Interestingly enough, Dr. Atkins was not always a proponent of what might be called mass-medicine, since publishing a book cannot be considered treating people on an individual basis.

In the January, 1966, issue of *Harper's Bazaar* an article appeared which talked about Dr. Robert C. Atkins, who was then a consultant in weight control to one of America's great corporations. His program advocated cutting down on carbohydrates rather than counting calories. This was much like his later advice. One difference stressed, however, was that since carbohydrate deprivation was "as potent in weight loss as the strongest medication . . . *uncontrolled* [my emphasis] it is dangerous and administered haphazardly it is worthless."

Atkins spoke of this regimen as needing to be "microregulated, fine-tuned by the doctor in charge." In other words, in order for it to be effective it had to be done with a physician. At the time that article was published, Dr. Atkins was apparently treating obesity on a "completely individual, custom-tailored" basis.

One has to wonder when Dr. Atkins began to believe that the individual treatment was not crucial and simply following the instructions in his book would suffice. He apparently changed his opinions about fat, too.

Part of the appeal of the Atkins Diet Revolution is that it allows you all the fats you want to eat. In the early days, Dr. Atkins came out against what was then called the Air Force diet, which encouraged the overuse of fat. That, Atkins felt, was "potentially dangerous because of its tendency to raise the serum cholesterol, thereby increasing the risk of heart disease."

In those days Atkins seemed to be diametrically opposed to the very sort of program he later dubbed a "revolution."

But, since our discussion is devoted to what is new in the field of diets, we ask whether there is anything new about the Atkins Diet Revolution. The answer is no. The best guess is that it was originated in the 19th century by a British surgeon William Harvey who, in turn, borrowed from a French doctor, Claude Bernard. The first recorded dieter using this method was William Banting who was so pleased with the weight he lost he published *Letter on Corpulence* in 1864.

In modern times it surfaced as *Calories Don't Count* by Dr. Herman Taller. Taller prescribed soft polyunsaturated fats as a stimulus to the liver to convert fat into energy. Taller's big mistake was in promoting the sale of safflower oil along with his book—for which he was sent to jail.

It seemed he specified a specific brand of safflower oil capsules that was made by a company in which he had a financial interest.

None of the above impresses me as much as one fact:

this diet may not work. You might not lose weight. And let's not forget the possible dangers of consuming too much fat.

A variation of this diet is the High-Protein diet, like *The Doctor's Quick Weight Loss Diet* co-authored by Dr. Irwin Stillman and Samm Sinclair Baker. That one could fit on one side of an index card, although you probably bought a book describing it. I did too.

Essentially, you can eat as much as you want of foods that are high in protein but this time, they must be low in fat as well. So you eat lean meats, poultry, fish, seafood, eggs and lowfat cheeses. Along with the food, you must drink six to eight glasses of water each day. The water is "to wash away the ketones."

It has never been established that high-protein regimens burn calories any faster than any other diet. Moreover, according to a Harvard medical study published in the *Journal of the American Medical Association,* too much protein can produce increases in blood cholesterol.

Another danger is in the directions: "Eat all you wish of these foods to satisfy hunger." Ahh, there's that old promise. Remember my good friend, Bill Gaines? It takes a lot more food to satisfy his hunger than mine. And there are plenty of times when I can consume as much as Bill and still not be "satisfied."

I tried Dr. Stillman's water diet, as *The Doctor's Quick Weight Loss Diet* was known. It seemed so simple. Nothing to think about. I could eat lean chicken, fish, cottage cheese. You are also permitted to use common seasonings such as salt, pepper, garlic, cocktail sauce, horseradish, ketchup, herbs and spices. There's no limit or directions on how much to use of these items. You can imagine how creative you become with your condiments; they soon begin replacing the foods they are supposed to accompany.

Conclusion? The diet, if it works at all, does so because you are so bored, you are ready to scream at the thought of another mouthful of anything lean.

But the water is really the topper. If you plan to try this diet stick close to home, or plan your traveling so you can get to a restroom frequently. I ended up dubbing this one "Stillman's Revenge."

Stillman was a great promoter of his book and became a familiar face on the television screen. His co-author went to work with the late Dr. Herman Tarnower whose Scarsdale Diet soon had countless people carrying around little plastic bags of spinach and dry protein toast.

The Scarsdale Diet was published in newspapers and magazines before it became a book. This one took up the space of one sheet of paper. Thanks to the writing talent of Samm Sinclair Baker, a page was turned into a book.

The regime, according to Dr. Tarnower, is "based on chemical reactions between foods rather than quantities of food." Simply stated, you are to use lean meat only, prepare foods without adding fats, use lemon or vinegar on salads and are permitted no substitutions! You must follow the day-to-day food plan strictly.

According to some medical observers the Scarsdale Diet is simply another low-carbohydrate, low-to-moderate-fat and high-protein diet. Although you don't count them, the calories add up to somewhere between 1,000 to 1,600 per day.

What makes the Scarsdale Diet effective is not eating two lamb chops on Wednesdays or cold chicken for Thursday's lunch. It works because you have reduced your intake of calories even if someone else has done the counting. That is why you are told to eat *exactly* what is assigned, with no deviation.

According to Toby Cohen, writing in *New York* magazine (May 21, 1979), the Scarsdale Diet, like similar ones, "manipulate[s] your eating habits. . . . it gets boring eating the same foods so you eat less; [and] the foods allowed by the durable all-you-want-of-this-but-not-that diets do not attract people who tend to binge." If that's true, it would indicate that for you bingers this probably wouldn't be an effective program.

The Scarsdale Diet cautions you not to go on it if you are a cardiac patient and to limit your use to no more than fourteen days at a time. And again, you are permitted to eat "plenty of steak" leaving *you* to make the decision as to how much is plenty. Many people left to their own decisions easily gained weight on the Scarsdale Diet.

According to Dr. Alvin N. Eden, writing in *Family Weekly*, "The unlimited quantity of steak allowed on Tuesday and Sunday seems rather strange. A one-pound steak contains 1,600 calories. You can readily see that a steak lover would have a difficult time losing any fat at all on those two days—all his weight loss would be water loss, a total waste of time and effort."

Like the high-fat diets, the Scarsdale offers a food program with high quantities of beef and the elimination of polyunsaturated fats. (You are not permitted vegetable oil or fat or butter and margarine.) We are left wondering about its nutritional wisdom.

The Scarsdale Diet has probably helped lots of people lose some weight—temporarily. But many physicians are wary. Dr. Peter Lindner, president of the American Society of Bariatric Physicians, feels that "the effectiveness of any approach must be measured in terms of whether there will be a reduced weight in 3–5 years, rather than 3–5 weeks or even months."

Dr. Lindner adds, "Only a gradual change in lifestyle, which will include better eating and activity habits, will have any long-lasting impact."

The Scarsdale Diet may get you to lose some weight but what about afterward? This is attended to in the "Keep-Trim Diet" section. Although the book talks about the great variety of "fine foods you may enjoy," there is also a rather extensive list of "All-Important *Don'ts.*" These include "*Don't* eat candy or chocolate. *Don't* eat spaghetti, macaroni products, noodles, other flour-based foods. *Don't* eat ice cream, ice milk, frozen custard, sherbet, or any frozen products that contain sugar or milk fats."

Never?

If the Scarsdale Diet is supposed to teach you how to eat for the rest of your life, I can see why people get fat again—and quickly—after they've gone off the program.

In order for any diet to work for you and for you to

keep thin, you must understand why you eat and you must learn to handle your food needs in a way that doesn't make you feel you are depriving yourself.

I can't imagine *never* eating ice cream. Can you? If you can, maybe you'll stay thin with the Scarsdale Diet. But don't fool yourself into believing it's a "new" diet. It's still basically only a 1,000 calorie a day program. Save your money and decide for yourself which thousand calories you want to eat, if that's the way you decide to reduce.

Why is it important to become aware about food? Why not just go on the next fad diet and follow it down the line?

Awareness is important because once you start making your own food decisions, you won't be an easy target for every "new" diet book that hits the bookstalls.

Becoming aware means giving up your belief in fairy tales.

We are all gullible to some extent. Every fat person wants to believe in the miracle cure that may appear one day. That gullibility is too often used to manipulate fat people by running false and misleading advertisements.

In *The Health Robbers*, S. Barrett and G. Knight point out that "most people frequently think health claims must be true or somehow they 'wouldn't be allowed.'" But I'll bet you didn't know that a false claim is against the law *only* if it appears in an advertisement or on a product label or is made in connection with a sale.

Forget miracles. There are none. Only hard work and

good common sense. Wouldn't it be nice if my friend
Wally's dream could come true? Wally always wished
he could eat everything he wanted without gaining
weight. "If only," he would dream, "they could insert a
tube that led out from the side of my throat so I could
eat and enjoy the taste of it and then just have it pass
through the tube."

Sorry Wally. And sorry all the rest of you. No tubes
this week.

We all think the next guy is a little weird when he
comes up with an idea like that one. But weird is in the
eye of the beholder. I guess the intestinal bypass operation looked pretty weird at first. Maybe Wally's wish
has been made possible by simply cutting off part of
your intestines!

Before you go rushing to your surgeon for a bypass,
(jejunocolostomy) understand that this is strictly a last-
resort strategy. It is to be considered only after everything else has failed. And, the side effects are possible
anemia, lack of calcium, and salt imbalance.

A recent issue of *Obesity/Bariatric* magazine describes one fifteen-year-old girl who'd had bypass surgery and later developed a problem absorbing vitamins.
Still another patient needed to reenter the hospital
within two months after the bypass surgery because of
an attack of gout.

Unfortunately, the second patient died. The autopsy
revealed kidney disease and pulmonary emboli (clots)
among other ailments.

The article suggests that before bypass surgery, the

benefits should be weighed against the possibility of other diseases arising due to the bypass itself.

Clearly, it's a drastic step. Moreover, there is growing evidence that bypass patients can and do regain the weight they lose.

If the bypass operation were not drastic enough, have you ever heard of a lipectomy? It is the surgical removal of fat. Right. They cut it out. If it sounds at all tempting, bear in mind it is done only when the person is so obese, as Drs. Elting and Isenberg describe in *You Can Be Fat Free Forever*, "they no longer can lie down to sleep since they have difficulty breathing in that position. . . . the weight of fat in the abdomen pushes the intestines up against the diaphragm, preventing it from moving properly."

What exactly is done? Excess fat is literally cut out of the body using an operating table that resembles a spit, in order to turn the patient around during surgery. Postoperative care involves watching for internal bleeding and heart or kidney damage. And, of course, there's lots of pain.

By the way, if this description isn't enough to make you lose your appetite, here is one further detail. The patient described by the above doctors was having the operation performed for the third time!

Shall we continue with more of the bizarre methods?

Some years ago there was a popular machine called the Relaxicizor. The impression was given that electrical current running from the machine to your body made the muscles contract and ultimately firm up.

One federal judge, upon hearing testimony on it, decided it might cause heart failure as well as possibly
exacerbate "epilepsy, hernia, multiple sclerosis, spinal
fusion, tuboovarian abcess, ulcers and varicose veins."
Well, anyway, the Federal Drug Administration put the
Relaxicizor on the prescription list.

I recalled what I'd read about the Relaxicizor when I
found an article in *Us* magazine (August 21, 1979)
about the Biobody Machine. This machine was discovered by Sasha and Joanna Muniak during their honeymoon in Hong Kong. The machine was used in Japan
on hospital patients for muscle therapy. The Muniaks
now use it in their Biobody Center to stimulate muscle
contraction. The article suggests further that "a 35-
minute session aimed at specific trouble spots, such as the
abdominal area, can equal 1500 sit-ups."

Hmmm. Has the Relaxicisor been reincarnated?

No concept is too farfetched for someone, somewhere,
who is desperately reaching for relief from the fat syndrome. That is why educating yourself about the real-
ities of various reducing programs is important. If you
learn the validity of the programs, you'll be able to
make your own, intelligent decision.

Anything magical, avoid. All magic is illusion, no
matter how well-performed. You want to achieve a long-
term weight loss, not one that will encourage pounds
to reappear like the rabbit in a magician's hat.

Why is it that magic always makes me think of hyp-
nosis? Many people have tried that too. For some it has
been known to help for a while. But since you aren't
learning anything about how to eat, or why you eat,

once the hypnotic suggestion wears off, you know by now what happens.

Not long ago an approach was introduced using the principle of acupuncture. In this instance, a special type of staple was permanently implanted in the patient's ear. Whenever unwanted eating seemed imminent all one had to do was stimulate the staple in a certain way and that activated nerve impulses which ended the desire to eat.

Sounds good. It was unsuccessful for an interesting reason. In order to make it work, the person had to stimulate the staple, and in many cases they just didn't do it. You see, nothing—even the most foolproof method —will work all the time. *You must want it to work.*

Remember cellulite? If you are female you probably have heard of and, Lord knows, feared cellulite. Cellulite, we were led to believe, is fatty tissue deposited in certain areas of the body—specifically the thighs, but also often on the upper arm.

There really is no such thing as cellulite according to Dr. Willibald E. Nagler, physiatrist in chief of New York Hospital at Cornell Medical Center. The word, taken from the French meaning "leather reinforcement on riding breeches," is "meaningless." Dr. Nagler says that the only way to get rid of this fat is by reducing caloric intake and by doing a great deal of aerobic exercise (swimming, jogging or running, bicycling, jumping rope, walking—briskly).

Best of all, keep your weight down and your muscles strong and you may not get it at all.

If it were only possible to reduce where we would

like! Dr. Donald S. Robertson of Scottsdale, Arizona, says, "I always explain to patients that we do not have much control over exactly where body fat will be lost, and that many times in order to get rid of abnormal thigh and abdominal deposits of fat [read: cellulite], we sometimes have to lose more total body fat than is desired, and the face and arms may become wrinkled in this process, but the undesirable fat will also ultimately disappear."

Apparently one way to get rid of "cellulite" is to diet enough to lose those fatty deposits. "Cellulite" is simply fatty tissue, no different from any other fatty tissue. Don't fall prey to the gadgets advertised that lead you to believe fat can be scrubbed away.

Whether you have contemplated bypass surgery or have merely been irked by the presence of "cellulite" on your body, you are not alone. Many hundreds of thousands of people have been ripe for the misleading promises of instant thinness.

None of these methods are solutions to your weight problem. *You* have the solution, and are now acquiring necessary knowledge about what works and what does not. And you are now ready to accept responsibility for your own weight problem.

Once you take responsibility for making yourself fat you can take responsibility for making yourself thin, also. The nice part of that is you can take *all* the credit for your success. You don't have to thank Dr. Stillman, Dr. Atkins, or any other doctor or diet you read about.

Weight control does involve giving up a lot of infantile behavior. But the rewards are more than worth it, believe me.

I know it is not easy to give up on miracles. A man I interviewed is probably the perfect example of the kind of person who will spend twice as much time and money looking for magical solutions than it would take if he tried to lose weight sensibly.

A few years ago he was desperate. He learned of a "new" diet. It entailed daily visits to a physician's office where he was injected with something called HCG or Human Chorionic Gonadotrophin. This is derived from the urine of pregnant women. The regimen was described by A. T. W. Simeons, M.D., in *Pounds and Inches: A New Approach to Obesity* published in 1972 in Italy. Dr. Simeons claimed that "the injection of only 125 units per day [of HCG] is ample to reduce weight at the rate of roughly one pound per day, even in a colossus weighing 400 pounds, when associated with a 500-Calorie diet."

Okay. So this fellow showed up every day at the doctor's office, dropped his trousers and bent over for his shot. The nurse (he rarely saw the doctor after the initial visit) handed him his food for the rest of the day.

At the end of the prescribed period of time he had lost a great deal of weight. It also cost him a lot of money. (Pregnant women's urine does not come cheap!)

He never once considered that *anyone* eating 500 calories a day would lose weight, with or without the injection.

Dr. Simeons talks about how long the treatment

should last. "Patients who need to lose 15 pounds (7 kg.) or less require 26 days treatment with 23 daily injections. The extra three days are needed because all patients must continue the 500-Calorie diet for three days after the last injection. This is a very essential part of the treatment, because if they start eating normally as long as there is even a trace of HCG in their body they put on weight alarmingly at the end of the treatment."

There is no way you can eat only 500 calories a day for twenty-six days and not lose weight.

But all the people who paid their money and dropped their pants didn't want to hear that. They were looking for the miracle. And even if they hated getting those shots, they held still for them.

I wonder how many kept their weight down. I know this man did not. Once he was on his own again and had no shots in the buttocks and no nurse handing him food, he had to make selections. And he was back to square one again.

Few of us want to hear the truth which, in this case, is that there is no evidence to suggest that HCG should work. It's the 500 calories you eat as opposed to the thousands you usually eat that makes you reduce.

The February, 1980, issue of *Consumer Reports* relates that "in a well-controlled clinical trial reported in the Journal of the American Medical Association, HCG fared no better than a placebo. Although HCG frequently has been prescribed to stimulate fertility, it has never been approved by the U.S. Food and Drug Administration as safe and effective for weight control."

Fact: Any "crash" diet can result in weight loss. The

above works, as we learn, because anyone who eats 500 calories a day is going to reduce. The rest of it is the stuff dreams are made of.

As Gilbert Leveille, Chairman of the Department of Food Science and Human Nutrition of Michigan State University, expressed it, "You can lose weight on just about any diet if you stick to it, but a fad or crash dieter will tend to stop and start diets often in the course of a year or two and ultimately gain five or ten pounds."

Did you read those last six words? Do you recognize yourself somewhere in that statement? What is there about us foodaholics that wants to believe in every fad, even though we know, somewhere within us, that there is no real miracle diet? Unless we learn to change the way we eat, we will lose and then gain again. No fooling.

Ah, but hope springs eternal.

I guess the ultimate dream may lie in an item just around the corner. Fake fat. Technically called sucrose polyester (SPE) this is supposed to help reduce and lower blood cholesterol.

SPE was synthesized by Fred H. Mattson, Ph.D., while he was a research scientist at Proctor & Gamble. (Now he is the head of Lipid Research Clinic at University of California in San Diego.)

SPE is supposed to imitate food fats in texture and taste, but—it is not broken down by the intestine and not absorbed by the body. (Be on the alert all of you who want to lose weight but cannot give up mayonnaise.)

SPE is calorie-free. It "binds to cholesterol on its way

through the intestines and carries it out in the feces. The result? Your serum cholesterol level can be brought down."

Before you begin looking for this fake fat on your grocery shelves, remember, it has a few more years of testing to go. Then it will probably show up first as a prescription drug meant to lower cholesterol. Eventually it might be substituted, the experts say, for 500 calories a day of fat.

I would reserve judgment on this one. Why look for fake fat? Isn't it better to learn to live with less real fat?

FOUR QUESTIONS TO ASK YOURSELF

1. What was the last fad diet you went on?

2. How much weight did you lose?

3. How long did you keep the weight off?

4. Are you ready to give up on fads?

If the answer to the fourth question is "Yes," you're ready to proceed. Otherwise read this chapter again.

Sabotage—or, What to Do About the Enemy?

Do you know what I'm talking about when I mention the enemy? I touched on this earlier when I told you about my sister, Jane. Jane, who was chronically overweight, had a husband who seemed determined to keep her that way. Anytime she had to lose weight, he would feel threatened that he might lose her and so, he did everything he could do to sabotage her weight loss plans.

This is not unusual. As a matter of fact, it is more commonplace than most of us are aware. When people who are trying to reduce share their experiences with others, one hears the frequent comment that those people who say they want to help us, really work against us.

The most obvious situation is that of parents who believe they are being thoughtful when they urge the child to eat that special dessert "only this once." At times like these, the dieter is frequently made to feel guilty for *not* eating.

161

I'm sure you have all heard things like "But I spent all day cooking this, and now you're not even going to taste it?" All too often cleaning your plate is interpreted as giving love to the person feeding you.

How many of us have eaten foods to avoid hurting other people's feelings? Plenty.

These feeding-friends are misguided. A true friend is one who encourages you in your effort, not one who complicates your problem.

In an article published in *Obesity/Bariatric Medicine,* a case was described where a patient had managed to maintain a 75 pound weight loss for a year and a half. Ironically, since the weight has come off, his family and friends greet him with: "Have you gained any weight yet?" I don't have to tell you that this is not the most helpful of questions to ask a person trying to stay thin.

First, the patient had to reassure himself that it was *their* problem, not his. He wasn't giving any cues to provoke this question. He also had begun to realize that he should not respond emotionally to what others think, say or do.

It's very difficult when you are seeking encouragement, and are not getting any, to hold on to your new thin image. It usually is necessary to analyze why people say the things they do. For one thing, don't dismiss the "sour grapes" attitude that so-called friends sometimes have.

It's like the old saying, "I want my friends to do well, but not so well that they do better than I."

It would be lovely to live in a perfect world, where everyone responds to us just as we would like, but if the world were perfect, we probably would not have the weight to lose in the first place.

A woman I know who lost a great deal of weight found herself reevaluating many friendships, especially those of her "friends" who had cautioned her against losing "too much weight."

It's sad, but a friend who is jealous of your success in getting thin and more attractive isn't a friend at all. That is a person who needs to feel superior to the people around him or her in order to feel adequate. Give such people up and seek new relationships.

Ironically, losing a great deal of weight is very much like becoming a new person.

If you realize that other people are not accustomed to dealing with you in your changed form, you can better understand that they need to adjust to this metamorphosis, just as you do. This doesn't excuse their counterproductive gestures, but might give *you* insight into possible motivation for such actions.

It's difficult to imagine people sabotaging your efforts, when it should be obvious to them how important their help is to your success. However, human interaction is quite complicated.

In *People Around You Can Make You Fat* Lee Headley, Ph.D., describes a man who had weighed 490 pounds and lost 238 of them. At the time of the writing he was trying desperately to put the weight back on. Why? It seems his wife, for whom he was trying to improve his figure, left him, complaining that he had lost his sense of humor.

You and I might ask, "Who needs a companion like

that?" Obviously, to this fellow, she was more important to please than himself. He chose to blame himself as being awful to live with and soon felt he was "getting back to my old self now."

If that's true love, save me from it!

Tell your friends, loved ones and relatives: "If you really love me, don't feed me." But at the same time, remember, just as it was you who put the weight on, and you who are taking it off, it's your task to deal with this problem too.

(I don't know of a single case where someone put a loaded pistol to an overweight person's head and said, "Eat.")

Beware of feeders. Gently but firmly refuse their "kind offers" of food "just this once," if you have decided it's against your better interest. This is difficult, I know, and you will sometimes find yourself jeopardizing relationships. However, you must consider how thoughtless the other person is being in not considering you.

You can devise all sorts of methods to dissuade your friends from over-feeding you. Some people like to see everybody at a party with a drink. Don't fight it. Just hold a glass of club soda with a slice of lemon or lime and you'll blend in with the crowd.

At a dinner party, make sure you leave some food on your plate. Otherwise, they'll be eager to rush in with seconds. Or, if your are being pressed to "just take a taste" tell them you have an allergy to that food. You'll find that no one ever tries to feed you food that might bring on a rash!

Don't be afraid to be an eccentric. If you find yourself

overwhelmed with a tempting array of foods and don't want to blow your diet, announce loud and clear, "Oh golly, too bad. Today is the day I always fast." That way, everyone will be watching to see if you break down. It will make you even more determined to stick with your resolve.

Beware, too, of "friends" who tell you how drawn and even sickly you look after you have dropped some weight.

A man I know had lost more than 80 pounds and many people greeted him by telling him he looked awful. That's thoughtless. When a fat person loses weight his formerly round features become more slender.

This fellow had many people not only tell him how terrible he looked, but that he looked better fat!

If you are involved in a program such as Weight Watchers or Overeaters Anonymous, these groups can be particularly helpful at times when you feel acquaintances are trying to sabotage your efforts. As I mentioned earlier, it is the support system that such groups rely upon that make the dieter feel understood and motivated.

You may be thinking that you have problems enough trying to reduce. Who needs to add to these by having to understand the motivations of others? If you look upon this knowledge as a vehicle that ultimately works for your well-being perhaps it's easier to accept.

If you try to understand what motivates these saboteurs you will be more secure in what you are trying to accomplish. Moreover, you will begin to accept your own judgments of yourself rather than those of others.

Just because someone tells you that the weight you have lost makes your wrinkles stand out more, or that you looked better fat, doesn't make it true.

There are a few instances where people may genuinely be puzzled and even disturbed by your weight loss. Young children sometimes feel threatened by any change in a parent. Don't forget, to that child, you are not fat, you are Mommy or Daddy. And children think you are perfect just the way you are.

Moreover, children see the entire world as centered around them. Thus, your weight loss may make them worry about losing part of you or worrying about other things in their world changing.

In *The Psychologist's Eat-Anything Diet,* Dr. Leonard Pearson tells of one youngster who said, "You're not fat, Mommy. You're soft. Don't you change."

As Dr. Pearson advises, reassure your children. Point out that their bodies keep changing but that doesn't alter the family loving one another. Assure the child, too, that you will love yourself better when you are thin.

As they approach adolescence and beyond, though, an obese parent can turn from "perfection" into a source of extreme embarrassment to that same child. Don't be surprised to hear demands to "get thin please!" from your kids. They love you, all right, but will like you better if you don't stand out in a crowd because of your fat.

Which brings me to an important question: Will *you* love yourself better when you are thin? Don't answer right away. Because the answer may not be the obvious one.

In order to really love yourself better thin you should find out what it is that makes you fat. Deep in your heart, do you dislike yourself? Are you punishing yourself with your fatness?

INTERMISSION EXERCISE

Have you ever had a "good friend" encourage you to eat when *you* know it was the wrong thing to do?

Make a list of those of your family, friends and acquaintances who try to push food at you. This is your secret enemies list. Henceforth, you must be constantly on guard when you, anyone on the list and food are all in the same place.

Why Do We Eat?

Hungry?
Bored?
Anxious?
Angry?
Afraid?
Depressed?
You can add to the list, I'm sure. How often, though, do you ask yourself, "Why am I putting this into my mouth?"

I know I eat for all of the above reasons. And more. I eat when I'm frustrated. I eat when I don't want to get to the work that I know I must get done. As I write this book I find myself wanting to jump up and raid the refrigerator. Eating is a great way to avoid getting down to business.

I suppose the only time I *don't* think of eating is when I'm having sex or horseback riding.

But why do you and I eat under these circumstances —while someone else does not? I'm not going to psychoanalyze you. I'd like to help open the door to discovery. What is it that drives you into self-destructive eating? Once the door to self-understanding is open, it will be up to you to close it when you wish.

I told you in the beginning that I was never the heaviest person alive nor am I now the thinnest. But I have struggled with weight most of my life and I understand how difficult it is not only to lose weight, but to keep it off.

I consider losing weight an enormous effort. It's one I've gone through many times. And it takes so much energy that I never again want to get fat enough to face what I call a "real" diet—one that will take more than a day or two, or maybe three, to take off the pounds that creep back.

It used to be difficult for me to understand how people could lose 50, 60, 100 and even more pounds, and then gain them all back again. I wanted to shake them by the shoulders and tell them, "Dummy! Wasn't it hard enough to take off those pounds? Can't you see that you're getting fat again?"

Of course I was not aware then of the many and varied reasons people eat.

One reason people reduce and then get fat again is because they are honestly afraid to be thin. No, don't laugh. What will it mean to be thin?

For one thing, they won't be able to hide behind their fat any longer. They will be just like everybody else. They won't be able to wallow in self-pity and blame other people for making them fat. And they will also have to face life's failures and disappointments without having fat as an excuse. Forced to stand on their own and take responsibility for their own actions—growing up.

That *is* scary!

It has been observed that psychological disorders suffered by the obese are more likely to be caused by being overweight than they are causes for the overweight.

Don't think, though, that fat people are more likely to be neurotic. Dr. Albert Stunkard, a psychiatrist at the University of Pennsylvania, found, in a study of New Yorkers, "only a 'trivial' difference between normal-weight and obese people in the amount and degree of mental illness."

But normal weight people don't have the added problem that fat ones do after reducing. Dr. Jules Hirsch of Rockefeller University in New York observed that "when obese people lose a lot of weight, a large percentage of them become depressed and anxious. . . . Many such people feel 'deprived, left out, lonesome and empty in a global sense.' "

Does this ring any bells for you? If so, it's particularly important to learn about how *you* deal with food. If you don't understand the interaction between yourself and the food you eat you certainly will continue to ride the roller coaster of getting thin and getting fat again. I want you to break that pattern once and forever. You can, you know. It's within *your* control.

Have you ever observed how overweight people just can't seem to throw food away? They'll go out and buy their food, eat to their satisfaction, and then, unable to discard it, but not wanting to eat more, they'll offer it to a neighbor. A friend, Anne Griffiths, is the neighbor of a magazine publisher who is forever on a diet. She's getting fat on his leftovers.

Do you have the fantasy that if only you can get thin, all aspects of your life will change? Will all your problems disappear?

No and you knew that. While it is true that you will change—drastically—the change in the physical you does not automatically mean that all other facets of your personality will change too. You have to work on changing them, if that's your desire.

Weight-related problems may end once you are thin, but don't be staggered to discover that you still have trouble getting the kids off to school on time, or that the house still needs dusting. The fantasy fades for fantasy-lovers. To soothe themselves they begin to nibble again. And up, up, up goes the dial on the scale.

A woman I interviewed for this book lost more than seventy pounds after being overweight all of her life. Her goal was, at long last, within her grasp. Only twenty more pounds. She already looked great, although the additional twenty pounds would obviously make her a knockout. She began to falter as she approached her goal.

When she questioned herself she realized that deep in her heart she was afraid of being thin. Part of the reason was that during all of her fat adulthood people —even strangers—would stop her on the street or on an elevator and make remarks such as, "If you ever lose weight life will be yours," and "You'll have men dropping at your feet."

What happened as she got thinner? Neither of those things. In fact, life was pretty much as it always had been. Naturally, she was disappointed. Was it all worth it?

She had not prepared herself for anything less than a total revolution in her life. But the reality is that lots of people are thin. So what? Men don't fall at your feet just because you are of normal weight. You have to find some other means of attracting attention. You must compete on the same terms as everyone else. Unless you are able to understand that, losing weight *can* be a big letdown.

It's as if you have been working on something and when you are ready to unveil it, the world looks at you, slightly puzzled. Unless you discover why you eat and are clear in your own mind about why you are losing weight, you may put it all back on.

But self-knowledge and self-understanding can become barricades against doing it again. Knowing what it is that makes *you* put on weight, again and again, can finally work to keep it off.

When you lose weight to please yourself, you get your own positive feedback. You will like yourself better thin and won't need to depend on the reactions of outsiders.

Some of the ideas we've all had about fat may be off base.

Some fat people get a great deal of consolation from eating. If they are lonely or unhappy or under stress, out comes the dish of crackers and cheese.

According to Dr. Lee Headley in *People Around You Can Make You Fat,* the funeral feast probably was born of a desire to soothe discomfort and grief. "The after-funeral spread allows self-comforting and a shared social expression of pain and sorrow."

Food does comfort. Don't let anyone tell you otherwise. Sure it keeps us alive, but we've come a long way since the eating was primarily for survival. That's how it is in our western civilization.

Wandering in the aisles of a supermarket or driving past the fast food restaurants that polka dot our major highways makes it difficult to realize there is still starvation in many parts of the world.

Food was the first comforting factor in our infant lives, as our mothers nourished us. But the way overweight people use food for comfort is what sets them apart from others.

Fat people use food as a way of rewarding themselves. Although most heavy people think of having no control over themselves when they eat too much, in reality they actually are controlling the forces that bother them by feeding themselves.

Food as reward for getting a lousy job done, a consolation for feeling unhappy, for getting the grass cut— all these are neurotic uses of food.

Have you ever seen a trainer reward a chimpanzee for performing his task in a circus? Put yourself in the chimp's place—maybe it will shock you into realizing what you are doing with food.

Food can be a pleasure; it should be. But you are not a performing animal. If a chimpanzee were more intelligent he might not be rewarded with food; he might get a trip to Paris. You have the option of feeding yourself because you have completed a task, or using some other, more constructive reward.

How about shopping? I hate to admit it, because shopping is such stereotypical behavior for women. But I'm going to let you in on something I discovered about myself not too long ago. When I feel down, shopping gives me a lift. Good or bad, it's the truth. And I'll tell you something else, it's not fattening!

When I buy something to wear and it looks good on me it helps to keep me from eating. The reason isn't very complicated. It's because it pleases me to see myself in the new skirt, or sweater, etc., and if I get heavy, it just won't look good.

But it isn't only shopping for clothes that gives me that lift. I can get some of the same good feelings shopping for greeting cards, stationery, or a beautiful coffee mug. You get the idea. The point is, instead of being "good" to myself with food, I have found other ways to please myself.

Try to substitute some pleasurable experience for your food rewards. Do you like to play golf? The next time you feel you have completed a particularly arduous task, go to a golf course or a tennis court and enjoy. Or sign up for a dance class or French lessons.

How about giving yourself an hour in a sauna and a massage?

Indulge your pleasure-oriented fantasies. You'll find that you feel fulfilled even more than you were when you hid in your room and ate a bag of donuts. Or if money is scarce, run a tub of water and soak in some Ivory liquid.

Many people eat because they are angry. They are angry and cannot express that anger directly. How many times have you fought with your husband (or wife) or your kids or your parents and then found yourself in the kitchen?

Sometimes eating is an expression of both anger and control. Certainly, it's a distorted sense of control. But control all the same.

Wouldn't it be better to let off that steam where you know it belongs? Get angry aloud. Tell the kids off. Are you afraid people won't like you because you yell occasionally? Bottling up anger can lead not only to food binges, but to more and more suppressed feelings of rage. Picture a pot ready to boil over and you'll know what I mean. If you take the lid off, you diffuse the anger and you can deal with it in an appropriate manner.

First, of course, you must try to accept the idea that it's okay to be angry sometimes. Everybody gets mad, you know. And those who let it out right away don't go around on the brink of a real blowup. They are less likely to develop ulcers too!

If you eat when you are angry, who ends up being hurt by your rage? You do of course. Feeding yourself when you're angry isn't going to make you feel better. It isn't even going to console you. It may make you fatter. And that surely isn't going to lessen your anger, is it?

I'm aware that reading this may make perfect sense, but the next time you come home from work and find that Billy hasn't walked the dog, or done his homework, and the garbage is piled up because no one took it out —you may still find yourself eating instead of giving Billy hell.

Try—just once—to handle your anger differently.

By the way, are you aware that obese people are rarely seen overeating? I mean, you don't see them actually putting food in their mouths. I know that my sister, Jane, almost never finished the food on her plate.

I questioned others who had struggled with weight problems to see if this was unique. One man told me that after a lifetime of sitting at his family's table and being criticized for taking an extra piece of bread or a second helping, after hearing over and over, "Do you really need that?" he finally withdrew from eating publicly. He would wait until he was by himself and could satisfy his eating needs in peace.

For others, eating is an act of defiance. It is saying to those who constantly hammer away at you: "My eating is one thing you can't control!" But of course, who suffers but you?

I've been straight with you all the way so let me tell you something nobody talks about. You've heard of "will power." And when you don't stay with your regimen you chastise yourself for lack of "will power."

Where is that "will power" supposed to come from? Some mysterious place deep within you?

Applesauce.

You can't buy "will power" at Bloomingdale's or Marshall Field's. It doesn't grow in a rose garden. It doesn't rain from heaven. The fact is, it is like the Emperor's new clothes. *It doesn't exist,* except in our imaginations.

So-called will power has to be self-generated. It has to come from inside. And the problem is that the will power oil drill may work twenty-three and a half hours a day but there will come that time when you reach in for the will power and the pump is dry.

I've been much more successful with won't power. Yes, *won't power!*

I won't eat those chocolate cupcakes because I'm going to trade them off for the pleasure of feeling better and looking better. I'd love to eat those chocolate cupcakes but I know from experience that I won't like myself or feel particularly good if I eat them. So I'll trade off immediate pleasure for pleasure to come.

It's like the things people do with money. Some of us can't hold on to it. We spend for immediate pleasure. The result is often deep insecurity because we have no funds to fall back on. Contrast this with the person who allows for some pleasure but also makes a regular bank deposit.

Passing by things you'd like to eat with "won't power" is like putting money in the bank. You'll get all that pleasure to come—and with interest.

Changing diet habits isn't easy. For some people, it seems no matter how much they eat or don't eat, they stay fat or get fatter. My good friend Phyllis virtually has to stop eating in order to lose any weight. And even then it comes off in meager ounces while she hungers to lose pounds.

For those of us who used to think that "eat less, lose

weight" was gospel, I don't know if it comes as good news or bad news to learn that it often is harder for fat people to reduce than it is for those just looking to drop a couple of pounds.

Dr. Judith Rodin, a psychologist at Yale University, points out that "fat people produce higher levels of insulin, a hormone that promotes the storage of calories as fat. High levels of insulin also cause hunger and result in increased food consumption. The faster a person eats and the more calories and carbohydrates the meal contains, the more insulin is released creating a cycle of more eating and more insulin."

Translated into plain language: fat people have bodies that are out of synch and eat more because their bodies cause them to. To make matters worse, according to Dr. Jules Hirsch of Rockefeller University in New York, pound for pound, overweight people "need a third to a half fewer calories to maintain their weight than people of normal weight."

Ye Gads! That makes you want to throw the towel in, doesn't it? What's the point in trying? It seems as though there's just no way to succeed.

Not true. I point out these grim facts, not to discourage you, but to let you know, if you are suffering, it's probably with good reason. Once you understand that it *is* harder for you to lose weight than other people you will be reassured that you weren't going crazy after adding up your daily caloric intake and it came to 200 but you still hadn't lost any weight yet!

Knowledge is an important tool. Ignorance can only breed frustration and overeating.

Let's continue with the depressing part of the scenario.

Not long ago scientists investigated the phenomenon I've just described. Dr. John H. Karam, director of the Metabolic Research Unit of the University of California at San Francisco, found that fat people either have a normal number of fat cells and these have become enlarged because they eat more calories than are used up, or they have *too many* fat cells and these, too, are enlarged.

I mentioned earlier that the number of fat cells a person has is determined during childhood. It is therefore terribly important to not overfeed children since infancy and adolescence are two periods in a person's life when the greatest amount of growth occurs.

But what about those of us to whom this information comes a number of years too late?

Despair is nonproductive. Learn to be realistic about your diet goals and about how long it may take you to lose weight. Understand your particular limitations. Before we part, I will help you to design a reducing program that will no longer frustrate you.

Brighten up! My approach is one you can embrace with no reservations because it will be one with reachable goals.

Do you have a morbid curiosity about discovering whether you are one of the "unlucky" ones? A physician can determine if you have high blood levels of insulin, triglycerides, and glucose, which could indicate that your fat cells are too big. If losing weight brings the three levels to normal, chances are the fat cells are down to normal size too.

Finding out isn't going to make you thin. But it need not diminish your determination to get thin. You may not be able to control the number of fat cells but you can control the size of them. If you are overweight and your blood levels are normal for insulin, triglycerides and glucose, it suggests that your fat cells are of normal size—even though they are too numerous.

Again, the focus here should be on reducing the stress connected with trying to get thin. *Don't allow yourself to get discouraged because it's going slow for you.*

I know how alone you feel when you start a new diet. But you couldn't be less alone. It has been estimated that some forty million Americans have serious weight problems. No, this information won't make you feel better; but at least you'll know that being overweight is not the loneliest game in town.

In the next chapters we're going to examine some of the commonly held myths about being overweight.

INTERMISSION EXERCISE

Why do you eat excessively?

Take a pencil and check the reasons below that apply to you. Then, number them #1, #2, #3 etc., in the order in which they start you overeating.

( ) Boredom   #__
( ) Anxiety   #__

( ) Anger   #__
( ) Loneliness   #__
( ) Depression   #__
( ) Frustration   #__
( ) Sexual frustration   #__
( ) Fear: specific   #__
( ) Fear: nameless   #__
( ) Love of food   #__
( ) Sugar syndrome   #__

Myths About Eating and Dieting

We all cling to certain excuses for why we are overweight. Probably the most common one is "I have a sluggish metabolism, and so no matter how I try, I can't ever lose weight."

Watch out, Pinocchio, your nose is going to grow!

Well, maybe that's not entirely fair. Maybe you really believe your statement. More than likely it isn't true. However, it is true that whereas most fat people start out metabolically normal, as they gain weight, research (done by Dr. Jerome Knittle of Mount Sinai Medical Center in New York, among others) shows that they may "gradually develop derangements in their internal chemistry." And, as these people may complain, this chemical derangement "can cause 'everything' they eat to turn to fat and result in weight gain even though they do not seem to overeat."

Another widely held myth is that fat people eat because they are emotionally disturbed. I've already quoted authorities who have concluded that psychological disorders are more likely the *results* than the cause of obesity.

And if you think you are fat because you inherited the "tendency," I do not offer myself as the only example that it is not necessary to fulfill that destiny. Studies of identical twins who grew up in different homes have shown that environment plays a stronger role than heredity.

In other words, if you have an inherited propensity to get heavy, you can stay thin if the environment in which you live encourages it. For those of us with such inherited tendencies obesity should be thought of as a chronic condition, one you can never forget, but one that can be kept under control.

Nevertheless, there are instances where physical problems are a very real part of the problem. Furthermore, if you have certain chronic conditions which require medical attention, these must always be taken into consideration before and during any weight-loss program.

Obviously, if you suffer from high blood pressure, arthritis, diabetes, or other special problems, you must work with a physician in selecting a diet program that will help you, rather than kill you!

But don't use a health condition to get off the hook, either. Obesity itself is a major factor in reducing your lifespan by leading to serious illnesses such as stroke, heart attack, gout, etc.

As for diabetes, Dr. Theodore B. Van Itallie, director of the Obesity Research Center at St. Luke's Hospital in New York, makes a persuasive case for losing weight. He says, ". . . Often, if you simply reduce, you can bring your blood pressure down to a satisfactory level and get diabetes under control."

If you have a special health problem, never, never go on a diet until you consult a physician.

Incidentally, obesity is not restricted to humans. Many people jokingly point out that after a period of time of living together, people often begin to look like their pets. An English study observed that "the pets of fat people are twice as likely to be fat as the pets of thin people."

That may sound funny, but if you have a dog like mine, it can be a real problem. Cinnamon is an apricot toy poodle, weighing about seven pounds. As I sit and nibble my cookie and sip my tea I find myself giving her the crumbs. It doesn't take very much overeating to make a seven pound dog fat!

Have you ever wondered if fat people are inactive because of or as a result of their weight? It gets hard to separate the chicken from the egg, doesn't it?

We've talked about exercise as an aid to weight loss. Let's talk about it for another minute. If you are very much overweight I doubt that you are the sort of person who would seriously embark upon a vigorous program of calisthenics, even if you can burn up 300 to 360 calories in an hour's workout. Nor would it probably appeal to you to take up skiing or paddleball, although you can expend 420 to 480 calories in an hour in those activities.

The fact is, you might just kill yourself too.

Once again, I recommend walking. Not only can you do it at any age, but it will tax your body far less for long periods of time than any other form of exercise.

Go for a walk. Take the dog for a walk. It will help the dog, too. Don't have a dog? Buy one. Or toddle over to your local Humane Society and get one, free.

We haven't yet touched on the effect of overweight on your sex life. On the most practical level, if you're extremely heavy you obviously limit your sexual flexibility. However, on an emotional level, I have spoken to fat people who confide that they are embarrassed by their bodies and tend to shy away from sexual contact.

In one such instance described in *The Psychology of Successful Weight Control* by Mary Catherine Tyson, M.D., and Robert Tyson, Ph.D., one young woman was advised by her doctor to lose weight. She knew losing would make her healthy and certainly improve her social life. However, she continued to eat as much as before and even gained weight.

When she discussed this problem with the physician, she admitted the fear of attracting men. She had been raised by strict parents and was taught that sex was distasteful. Her lesson was so well learned that she unconsciously avoided men by making herself physically unattractive. Thus, in her case, staying fat meant staying "safe."

Yet, in other cases, obese women may become sexually aggressive because, fully aware of their appearance, they have decided not to be overlooked by men. Instead, they go after men of their choice. Many, however, choose men who are sexually submissive and who ultimately do not fulfill them.

As far as sexuality goes, though, fat people are just as interested in sex as the next person. Don't delude yourself by believing otherwise. But it also may be true that sex drive can decrease because the added bulk you're carrying makes it more difficult to get around.

I hope it's clear that we are not eliminating either gender from this discussion. Men and women can be equally sensitive because of their body weight and have sex hangups.

During the period of life when men are passing through their climacteric (male menopause) they experience symptoms which are similar to those women encounter at menopause. Because hormonal changes are occurring, some men gain weight. With the weight gain they may feel their sexual powers leaving them. It's important for them to understand that sexual powers are decreasing not because of the "change of life" but rather, because they are getting heavy.

In *You Can Be Fat-Free Forever,* Doctors L. Melvin Elting and Seymour Isenberg describe one man who was having such an experience. After becoming thinner than he had been in thirty years, however, he found himself passing through the male menopause and emerging more sexually active than before. As he put it, "I've discovered there's a lot more still left to me in life than food."

A *Good Housekeeping* article discussed twenty-five of the most commonly believed myths about weight. I won't cite them all, but it's worthwhile taking a quick look at a few.

If you stay on your diet you will lose weight every week. The fact is, we all reach plateaus where no weight loss occurs. If you believe you *must* lose weekly pounds, it may throw you off course.

After dieting for a while, the stomach shrinks. (This is one I always thought was true.) The fact is if you reduce permanently the quantity of food you eat, after your weight is down for several months, you actually will feel full sooner, because you require less food. It's a matter of getting your body accustomed to the smaller quantities. Your stomach does not change size.

When I was much heavier, I can recall going with friends for our usual Sunday night Chinese dinner. There were four of us and we always ordered food enough for six. I think we believed we would have leftovers to take home, but there seldom were. As I lost weight I found myself amazed at how my capacity dwindled. I just could not consume the same quantity of food as I had earlier. Had my stomach shrunk? I thought so, until I learned the above.

I like to think that my body has outsmarted me. I put it that way because when I was reducing I always planned that when I got thin, I would always save room for desserts at dinner, no matter what. I'm a person who scans the dessert section of a menu first and then I decide what I will eat. Thus, if I see a tempting dessert I adjust my dinner to accommodate it.

Ironically, I often find myself too full to eat the dessert. Yes, *too full*. I never dreamed that could happen on my way down, but it has. I'll bet you don't think that will ever happen to you, either?

It will.

You need extra vitamins while you are dieting. We certainly are hammered at by television and radio as well as print ads to make us believe so. But if you eat a well-balanced diet, there is no need for vitamin supplements. Moreover, if you think you can go on a fad diet and supplement what your body is lacking by taking vitamins, that isn't going to happen, either.

I heard the strangest example of this attitude from a man who called in to one of those "talk" radio programs where the listener can speak to the "expert" on the air. This day the studio guest was a diet specialist who was also an expert in nutrition.

The caller had problem. He had devised a fad diet of his own. He ate dry cereal which came in single portion boxes. He did so because he could read the outside of the box and know exactly how many calories he was consuming. It also gave the vitamin breakdown. His question was, how many boxes of cereal did he have to eat in order to have a perfect quota of vitamins daily?

There was a long moment of total silence before the expert could respond that this was an extreme example of how people can misinterpret concepts!

Does alcohol stimulate appetite? Some people find that when they are tense their appetite may diminish (unless they are the type that eats out of control under the same conditions!). Since alcohol can relax you, it can also turn on your appetite by reducing tension. But then, any form of relaxation would help appetite come back; it doesn't necessarily have to be alcohol. Food also acts as a relaxant, which is one reason we eat when we're tense.

As all of us veteran dieters know, alcohol contains calories which you just have to tack onto your intake count. Most drinks contain more than 150 calories. It's important to understand how your body uses alcohol in order to judge whether it's worth eliminating or keeping it part of your life.

As described in *The Psychology of Successful Weight Control,* food, when eaten in large quantities all at once, is either used as energy or stored as fat. Alcohol, on the other hand, if taken in quantity at one time, is mostly converted into body heat or soon excreted. (So that's why I always feel the need to run to the bathroom after a few drinks!)

If you plan to drink, the authors of the above book suggest that you have it quickly and at one time, rather than spreading it out over a long period. Whether or not this is practical for you I'll have to leave to you to decide. You may, after all, find that drinking a large quantity of alcohol quickly will make you pass out. I'd take this advice with some caution.

My own experience with alcohol is that a little bit can take *away* my appetite. However, a little bit too much just turns on my munchies and off I go. I have to be very careful. And I'm not going to tell you how much is "a little bit" and how much is "a little bit too much," because it's different for everyone. Some people can put down five martinis and they have no effect. If I put that many drinks away, I'd be out like the light from a weak candle in a hurricane!

Have you always believed that eating just before bedtime will add pounds? The facts imply that *when you eat has nothing to do with gaining weight.* A calorie is a calorie, by day or night. It doesn't matter when you consume it.

I guess you've discovered from this section that many of the ideas people have had about getting fat and getting thin aren't true. They are nice, comfortable excuses we use to fall back on in order to not take responsibility for making ourselves stay overweight.

Once you give up the myths, you will more successfuly find solutions to getting thin.

EIGHT GAMES TO PLAY TO ADD STRENGTH TO YOUR ATTACK

1. Buy your favorite snack food. Take it to the nearest waste basket and dispose of it untouched.

2. Go to a restaurant and tell the waiter you are on a diet and to please serve you only half portions.

3. Take a long look at your favorite food that fattens and then imagine it as it will be after somebody digests it.

4. Make up an absolutely outrageous tale to tell to your companion at the next meal you share in a restaurant. Such as, "I can't

eat much. You see, I swallowed this diamond
and . . ."

5. Buy half a dozen grapefruit and make
them your entire food intake for the day.

6. Fast one day a week for the hungry
children of an Asian or African country and
send a check for the food you would otherwise
eat to a United Nations fund for those
children.

7. Prepare a large portion of one of the
foods that make you fat. Pour three tablespoons of liquid detergent over it. Now ask
yourself if you want to eat it.

8. Drink four glasses of water before
you take your first bite of dinner.

The Nitty Gritty— or, How to Get to Where You Want to Go

We've talked about why we eat. We've talked about our cravings for certain foods. We've talked about the emotional and physical aspects of the food that goes into our bodies. We've talked about some fairly well-known diets of recent years and how they may not be the most effective methods to reduce—*and to stay reduced.*

We've also discussed being realistic about setting a goal for your weight loss.

This information is your investment in you. You are now going to lose weight by making intelligent, realistic decisions in designing your own diet. The pounds you take off now can stay off, if you use your newly acquired insight.

This time it *is* going to be different than all the other attempts. You promised me, and more important, you promised yourself!

This time you are going to accept responsibility before-hand for making yourself fat. That way, you can also pat yourself (and only yourself) on the back when *you* have made yourself thin.

This time you are going to really examine your food needs from every angle. You are going to think about what foods you feel you just "can't live without." And, you are going to try to fit these foods into your diet plan. Remember, *there are no forbidden foods, only forbidden ways to eat.*

You are going to discover when are the hungriest times of the day for you. Not everyone agrees about the importance of eating three meals a day. To Dr. Nevin Scrimshaw, head of the department of nutrition and food science at M.I.T., "There is no natural law that requires two, three or four meals a day."

While it is important to maintain a balanced approach to eating, it is not important whether you eat two, three or many meals daily.

Dr. Scrimshaw further observes that "The frequency, pattern and time of meals, as well as which foods are appropriate at that meal, are culturally determined."

In some countries people eat a continental breakfast consisting of coffee or tea, a roll or pastry and maybe juice. Yet elsewhere it is traditional to have a large meal to start the day.

For me, the morning is the easiest time to go without food. I'm genuinely not hungry or interested in food in the A.M.

I can hear you saying, "You have to start your day off

with a good breakfast." Break out of that mold. There's no law that says you *must* start the day with eggs and bacon. Or cornflakes and milk.

I know that most overeaters are also breakfast skippers. But there is no straight line relating those two facts. If you believe breakfast will get you off to a good start for the day, have it.

I'd rather pass and here is my reason why.

I am no longer a growing girl. If I were a child whose body was still forming, I could understand the need for certain kinds of food during any single day. Even pediatricians now suggest that parents keep an eye on the overall food intake of children, rather than what is eaten in one particular meal, or even in one day.

For instance, if a child eats a great deal of candy or cake one day, he may compensate the next day by getting in those veggies and protein. At the end of a week, a "balanced" diet should have been consumed.

We no longer have to be uptight about scheduling our food. Most of us eat not because we are hungry; we eat because it's lunchtime or dinnertime. If you were put in a room where there were no clocks and you couldn't tell if it was morning or evening, you would have to rely on stomach time to tell you when to eat.

Thin people eat more according to "stomach time" than to other cues like odors, availability and the clock. Yes, thin people are different from you and me. They eat only as much as they need to satisfy their hunger. Then they stop.

A fellow I know is one of those thin people. Before

meeting him I had my own theory about thin people which was that most of them don't like desserts or similar foods that made *me* fat.

Then I met Buddy. Buddy is not only thin, but if he misses a meal he *loses* weight. He has to keep reminding himself to eat something or he just can't keep up his weight. (Hey, don't you wish that was you?)

I figured Buddy for one of those thin people who fit into my theory. I soon found out how wrong I was. Although some naturally thin people don't quite understand what all the fuss is about when people envy them, Buddy truly appreciates his station in life. Buddy's wife is like the rest of us; if she eats too much, she gains weight.

Buddy truly enjoys food, and especially desserts. He was particularly fond of a deep-dish strawberry pie which could be purchased only at a tiny bakery in Greenwich Village, New York. (Unfortunately for Buddy, it has gone out of business.)

When strawberry pie was available, Buddy made for the bakery and bought several. He didn't want to run short. He dug into those pies and ate and ate. But an interesting thing happened. Just as soon as Buddy was full (although because it was strawberry pie, he might eat more than usual) he put his fork down. Not because anyone told him to. He put down his fork because he just could not eat any more. It didn't matter whether there was pie left on his plate when he stopped.

The difference between Buddy and a fat person is that the fatty would keep eating until all the pie was gone.

Thin people eat to satisfy hunger, not appetite. They don't eat because their parents told them what good children they were if they cleared their plates. They eat because they are hungry. And, they can sometimes become so involved in activities, they forget to eat.

I'm not going to tell you that this will ever happen to you. It hasn't happened to me, and I've been thin for years.

It doesn't matter. What does matter, is realizing the difference between people who are struggling with obesity, and those who aren't.

Food has a different meaning for chronic reducers than it does for thin people whose focus is directed else·where. Some people, comparatively rare in number, are altogether disinterested in food. In my lifetime I have met only two, and I don't envy them.

Eating, after all, can be one of the great pleasures of life. It is for me and it will be for you too when *you* learn to control food rather than allowing food to control you.

To be totally fair, one of the two non-food people appears to like food very much. Captain J. Peter Moore was associated with Sir Alexander Korda and later, for about ten years, managed the affairs of the egocentric artist Salvador Dali.

Captain Moore happens to be an excellent cook and dines in the most elegant restaurants in the western world. However, once he has tasted the delicious food, he loses all interest. After a few bites he moves the food around on his plate so that, if you haven't watched carefully, you'd believe he is eating.

The other person truly dislikes food. Remember the

Jack Spratt nursery rhyme? That's her story in reverse. This woman is married to a food-obsessed fellow who is forever eating and forever trying to lose weight. When this couple married, he planned a gourmet honeymoon eating at all the four-star restaurants in Europe, not being aware of his bride's antipathy to food. The scenario was lively if not pleasure-packed.

If we can focus on someone who is thin without having to diet, and observe how that person eats, we will learn that they do many of the things I suggest in this book. But they do them naturally.

For instance, they finish swallowing what is in their mouth before putting more food into it. Between bites, they put their food down (if it's something you hold in your hand like barbecued chicken). They put down the fork while they are eating, rather than impatiently waiting to shovel in more food. Watch, you'll see I'm right.

I'm going to let you in on another bit of important information. Although I consider that I have won my war against overweight, even though the war is over, the mop-up battles never end.

I must constantly remind myself of priorities. Most of the time I operate pretty much on automatic, eating sensibly. But there are also times when I need to focus myself all over again. For instance, when I wrote the paragraph about watching how thin people eat, what I was saying seemed perfectly clear. Then I had an immediate opportunity to apply that advice.

The evening I wrote the paragraph I refer to, I had a dinner engagement. By now you know how much I like desserts. So naturally, I planned to leave room for a calorie treat. Dinner was enjoyable and I ate more than I planned of the main course. And, there just wasn't anything terriffc enough in the desserts offered for me to indulge.

Fine.

Later I got home and found one cookie I'd forgotten. It was sitting in the cupboard. I decided then that it would be dessert. As I ate it, I remembered what I had written about how thin people eat. I remembered how they don't stuff food into their mouths until they have finished what is already in it. They put the food down while they are chewing. And so forth.

I ate that cookie differently. I made it into an exercise on eating like a "thin" person. I took a bite, then put the cookie down and savored the flavor of what I was eating. The exercise proved to me that I could enjoy food without compulsively consuming it unthinkingly.

What I hope I am conveying to you is that I am constantly learning and relearning about food and myself. I never will feel I know everything I need to know about staying thin, because for those of us who have been fat and want to stay thin, food can *never* be eaten unconsciously.

Always remember: knowledge *is* power. And with adequate knowledge you will have the power to reduce and remain thin.

I guarantee it.

Realistic Goals

When I was at my fattest I swung back and forth
like a pendulum about weight goals. First I wanted to
be 100 pounds. It seemed like a nice easy number to
remember. At other times I felt it would be impossible
for me to lose more than ten, maybe fifteen pounds.

When you are heavy it seems impossible to become
what you believe is *really* thin. It's also difficult to accept anything less than a weight that is probably impossible to achieve.

Of course, by setting your goals this way it makes it
impossible to do anything, so you eat another sandwich
and think about it.

How do we set a realistic goal? First, I'll tell you how
not to set one. My girl friend used to watch the Miss
America beauty pageant each year. When they announced the measurements of each contestant, my friend
enjoyed comparing her weight to that of the young ladies

competing to become the number one popular symbol of physical perfection.

If that year produced a large number of ladies whose weight was close to my friend's weight she would rationalize herself out of trying to take off those pounds she normally believed did not belong on her body. "If Miss America and I are the same weight, I must be okay." (Naturally, she did not bother to comment on whether or not the weight looked different when it was distributed on Miss America. Or whether the potential Miss America was five inches taller than she was.)

We often set goals according to the measurements of people we admire. I can recall poring over magazine articles about some of my favorite movie stars which occasionally mentioned their weight. If it was a low figure I decided that if it was good enough for Miss Movie Star, it would be perfect for me.

I didn't consider how the movie star's weight would have looked on my frame.

Apart from the obvious juvenile manner of deciding on a goal, here is another reason why patterning your weight after someone else's is unrealistic.

I grew up admiring Elizabeth Taylor. I still believe she is one of the most beautiful women on earth. When she was young she could take your breath away. As she matured her beauty remained, but her body got out of hand. One magazine article mentioned her weight. It was a surprisingly low figure.

My God! If Elizabeth Taylor weighed *that* and looked considerably overweight what on earth did I look like, weighing ten pounds more!

When I read that article it never occurred to me that maybe the figure was not quite accurate. Maybe it was an affectionately written piece and thus understated her weight. I believed every word, especially about her weight.

Overweight people spend the greater part of a week getting on and off of the scale. Now we have digital scales which can tell us to the tenth of a pound how much we weigh. Were they trying to tell me that Elizabeth Taylor did *not* weigh in as was suggested in that article? Whom could I believe anymore?

And who really cares how much Elizabeth Taylor weighs? Except Elizabeth Taylor. Soon enough Elizabeth Taylor reached a point in her life when she decided to do something about her extra pounds.

If there is inspiration to be taken from her, it might be that she found an effective method of reducing, not because she reached a specific weight. Her weight has nothing to do with yours.

If you are curious about how she reduced, I'll tell you. She entered the Palm-Aire spa in Florida for three weeks of determined and disciplined hard work at exercise and diet. There was nothing unique about the program given to her at the spa; it was much the same salt-free diet most guests receive.

Ms. Taylor worked with the head of the medical staff, Dr. Alfred Moore, and the dietitian, Andrew Adriance. With the dietitian she discussed her eating habits as well as her attitudes about food. (In other words, she did exactly what *you* are going to do to reduce.)

I don't think it's of particular importance to tell you

what time she ate breakfast or what she ate for dinner. The point is, she accepted the fact that she needed to lose weight and she did something about it. That is what should inspire you about Elizabeth Taylor, not how much she weighed when she left the spa.

Few of us can afford the expense of going to a spa to reduce. But eventually even the people who can afford it have to leave the protective atmosphere. If you can learn how to handle food in the real world you'll have an advantage over those who have been pampered and reassured, but not prepared to maintain a thin life style alone.

How are you going to figure out how much you ought to weigh? The first step is to look at yourself as you are now. Get in front of a mirror naked. That's right, strip down to skin. Don't look away. This may be the first time you've taken a good look at yourself in a long time. Examine every inch. This is a critical look so don't expect that you are going to be thrilled with what you see.

Hold in your stomach. Nothing happens, right? Still there. Turn around and look at your rear too. Use a hand mirror and scrutinize your body slowly.

How long have you been in the shape you see? A few months? Years? Have you been carrying that excess weight ever since childhood? Did you put on weight during pregnancy and never take it off? Was your pregnancy fifteen years ago? Did you gain weight after you stopped smoking? When did you stop smoking? (My ex-husband used that excuse for two years!)

Now get dressed. The examination is over—temporarily. A grown person should only have to endure so much punishment.

Boy, are you lucky!

Yes, lucky, because you now have a clear-cut job to do that will bring you a great sense of accomplishment.

When you set your goal, think about the questions I asked. How long have you been fat? That's important. Because you must realize that you are not going to get thin overnight. *If you have been carrying around excess pounds for a long time you must set a goal that will insure success.*

In setting your goal be realistic about something else. Certain aspects about you can never be changed, no matter how much weight you lose. Your body type and shape are with you forever.

In 1940, Dr. W. H. Sheldon categorized all bodies into three types. The ectomorph is the guy who is long and lanky. The mesomorph is more rectangular or pear-shaped with sturdy arms and legs. The curvy endomorph is more rounded, tending towards the plump.

These type categories are now universally accepted. We all fit into one or another of them with some over-lapping. However, as long as you believe that losing weight is going to reshape your basic structure, you are headed for nothing but frustration.

To give you a different analogy, it would never occur to you to try to become two inches taller than you are. You accept your height because you know you can't change it, even if you'd prefer being taller or shorter. However, with your figure it's somewhat different.

It is true that when you reduce you eventually reduce everywhere. But I came to peace with myself long ago over the fact that no matter how thin I get, I'll always have thighs that are a little bit bigger proportionately than the rest of me. This is a fact of life it's best to learn to live with. It'll help you be happier about accepting yourself when you get to your goal.

If your goal is to lose one hundred pounds in two months you are not going to be able to do it. No way. But if you tell yourself that in one month you want to be eight pounds lighter, your chances are very good that you will succeed.

If you think eight pounds is not satisfactory for one month, you are getting impatient. And impatience is nonproductive. If you have a lot of weight to lose, develop the attitude that you are going to reduce in stages.

No one can lose one hundred pounds all at once. But if you figure out how much weight you will lose in one year if you reduce eight pounds each month, you'll discover that adds up to ninety-six pounds. (Pretty close, you'll have to admit.)

If you set your goal in that fashion you can succeed. How about a loss of as little as one pound a week? Nothing? It's a reasonable, manageable goal to accomplish. Losing four pounds a month is a snap. It's so easy you'll wonder why you struggled and agonized all these years. One pound a week? Of course you can do it!

Not fast enough, my fat friend? You want to raise your goal to eight or twelve pounds a month? Take heed. Have you been able to maintain any of the weight lost on crash programs? And if you had begun to lose a pound a week one year ago, today you would be *fifty-two pounds lighter.*

An acquaintance of mine who had been skinny most of her life suddenly was thirty pounds overweight when she discovered she had hypoglycemia. This condition caused intense sugar cravings, which she indulged.

Never having had to diet before, my friend went to her physician. He put her on a program which had her reducing very slowly. As a matter of fact, if she lost *more* than the one and one-half pounds a week, as prescribed, he adjusted her menu by adding food.

While you are setting this "easy" goal, remember too that there will be times when you will not lose weight. You are human, not a machine. You can't actually "walk off" a piece of apple pie by figuring out how many calories you "burn" by walking. Your body is too complicated a mechanism. But if your goal is one pound a week and you stumble one week, you'll catch up in the next stretch. It's reachable and healthy. Don't allow one brief failure to balloon into giving up and bingeing.

Very important.

What with premenstrual, menstrual and postmenstrual periods, women sometimes find themselves having more difficulty losing weight at different times of the month. Moreover, women can be extremely discouraged to discover a temporary weight *gain* from water retention at these times, even though they know they haven't been overeating.

It's important to plan for these times when you seem

not to be losing. If you know they are going to occur, you won't look at them as setbacks because they will be part of your plan.

For instance, if I were setting my goal and it was four pounds a month, I'd go one step further. I would remind myself, perhaps by writing it on a calendar, that when my period was due I would not lose weight and might even show a gain.

The menstrual cycle is not a constant either. There's no guarantee that each month you will retain fluids around that time. Sometimes it happens and sometimes it doesn't. However, if you *plan* not to lose during that time, you can only feel delighted if you do drop weight.

It's all part of the little game we learn to play with ourselves. You must never ever kid yourself, but you can learn to pretend or just not pay attention and then be pleased with a positive result.

To go even further, during the time just prior to and during my menstruation, I would determine not to get on the scale. This is difficult. There is a thin line separating positive and negative motivation and only *you* know when you've stepped across it.

There are times when I know my weight is up and then I decide to weigh myself. When I make the decision it's because I know that seeing the number will startle me into getting the weight off. However, there are other times when I know my weight is up and I will not go near the scale. I know that those are times when weighing myself will not be productive but might make me depressed enough to eat. So, I avoid the scale.

Get to know your body and your psyche. Discover the days when you seem to have more difficulty reducing. Get an overview by comparing one month to another. See if you can't establish a pattern that will give you insight. If you accomplish this you will not only lose weight, you will feel very much in control of yourself. You won't think some outside forces are working against you, making it difficult to lose.

Even if you don't have fifty-two pounds to lose set your goal with the future in mind. If you want to lose twenty pounds use the same principles. Don't expect to lose all the weight at once. Don't even try. *Don't* crash diet. The pounds you lose on a crash diet will not stay off!

Break that pattern of three days eating and three days dieting. This time, keep in mind your promise to be realistic, whether it's one hundred pounds, twenty pounds or five pounds. You are not going to lose fast and repent slowly this time.

Plateaus will occur when you won't seem to lose any weight. A plateau is a time when your body is readjusting to your new weight. There are times when your weight won't budge. You can actually learn to enjoy the plateau and make that period a positive one. After all, you are thinner than you were, so you can congratulate yourself for accomplishing that.

Learn to use plateaus to your advantage.

Marking your calendar and plotting your weight loss can keep you in touch with your over-all success. The finish line is always surprisingly near.

As you approach that line, prepare yourself to enjoy and accept your new figure. Learn to accept the compliments you are going to receive. Resist the temptation to tell everyone how fat you used to be.

Teach yourself to be delighted with the new you. Be content with your chosen goal if it is still reasonable. Be aware of the danger at this point of trying to reduce more than you believe you really need to. Don't become a compulsive dieter.

Now you know how to select your goal. Whether it's 150, 200, 40 or 10 pounds. You have determined how much you need to lose. You've taken out your calendar and marked down how much weight you expect to lose as well as the realistic rate at which you expect to go down. You promise you're not going to get any thinner than your goal.

There's yet another important step.

Make time for more introspection. Yes, you still have to learn more about yourself so that you can decide just which approach will be especially helpful in your individual weight loss program.

Get to know yourself and forget why your neighbor seems to be losing when she also seems to be eating pizza all the time, while you subsist on what seem to be starvation rations.

She isn't you. And you aren't her.

Leave your ego in the closet and accept the opinions and comments of your friends as well intentioned. Pick someone you love and trust, whom you know feels the same about you. Thus, you won't interpret your friend's observations as criticism.

Pay particular attention to what triggers eating. Do you find yourself getting up from your chair at every television commercial and hitting the nibbles? When I come home from work, immediately after I hang up my coat I head for the kitchen.

It's quite normal for people to be hungry in the late afternoon or early evening. After all, it's been several hours since lunch and it's not quite dinnertime. It's actually *danger time*.

If you know this is your pattern make up your mind to change it by not going to the kitchen. Instead, go directly to the bathroom. Don't even put your coat away. Brush your teeth. This activity will act to clean your palate and give you the time you need to make a conscious decision about whether or not you want to go into the kitchen.

If you can't do this, and find yourself in the kitchen, prepare foods that will be on hand for immediate grabbing. These should be foods and beverages that won't add weight.

You might find that the refrigerator is not your enemy. Instead, the villain may be the pantry where you stash the crackers or potato chips.

I deliberately move these to the top shelf so that to reach them I must climb a stepladder. The moment's interval between climbing and reaching often makes all the difference for me to become acutely aware that this is not what I want to be doing.

I keep certain foods in the refrigerator which are the first thing I see when I open the door. These are carrot sticks, celery, radishes, etc. They may not nourish my spirit, but they do my figure just dandy.

The above hint was offered to me by personal nutrition counselor Carryl Atton who is based in New York City. Her expertise is in behavior modification. She works with people on a one-to-one basis to help them analyze their food needs, manage their goals and modify their eating behavior.

You have eaten the way you do and it makes you fat. If you don't change that, you will get fat again. People who lose weight on liquid protein are learning nothing about their relationship to food and the world. Unless they learn, zoom, on go the pounds. Eating bananas and milk for a month will make you lose weight. So will Grape Nuts cereal and an apple, three times a day.

Even a one-sided diet like ice-cream-only will result in weight loss. But are you prepared to spend the rest of your life sipping liquid protein or eating bananas and milk? Any weight reduction program must include foods you feel you can eat over an extended period of time.

You can plan your own program which will be quite different from the next person's. Don't forget, no food is forbidden. It's the way it's handled that you have to watch.

I eat better now than I ever did when I was fat. When I was fat I was nondiscriminating about food. I am very selective now because I know I'll get fat again if I return to my old habits. Once you have developed better food habits and learn to enjoy food it's difficult to be satisfied with junk.

Snobbish?

Maybe.

But it works for me.

Let's determine what will work for you.

WINNING THE RESTAURANT GAME

1. Never eat in a restaurant that offers an "all you can eat" buffet

2. If there are bread and butter on the table, ask the waiter to remove them

3. Order à la carte (Don't order a "complete lunch" or "complete dinner.")

4. Once in a while, order two appetizers and skip the main course

5. Be the last person of those at your table to start eating

Some Observations
on Motivations

Some insurance companies are becoming aware that they can motivate people to lose weight.

The September 1979 issue of *Inc.* magazine described how the Admar Group, a Santa Ana, California, insurance company, proposed a contract where employees agreed to participate for a year and try to lose at least fifteen pounds.

Employees have an option of taking behavior modification classes at a local hospital. If they lose the minimum number of pounds (there's no maximum limit), the fee for the course is reimbursed by the company. And for each pound of weight they lose, the company pays them $3!

It would be marvelous if more companies became involved that way. But until they do, you can rely on the group efforts of such organizations as I've mentioned. Don't forget, though, that it's still up to you in the end.

There are people who think they are accomplishing something positive by taking diuretics to help them reduce. Diuretics help excrete excess water our bodies may hold from time to time. These are frequently used by women during that bloaty time of their menstrual cycle.

As long as you are aware that it's water you are losing and not fat, you're all right. I know, I know. Who cares what is coming off as long as the scale indicates a loss? I understand that feeling. But if you depend upon water loss to get thin, you will be discouraged after you have gotten rid of all excess water and there's still the hard work of getting rid of the fat.

Always remember that the diuretics are *aids* to your reducing plan, if you decided to use them. But they cannot accomplish anything without your help.

There is the danger of losing potassium while taking diuretics so be sure to consult a doctor before using them. He may want you to supplement what your body may be losing, or he may prescribe one which has potassium added.

Finally, if you have a high uric acid count, diuretics can raise it dangerously and trigger the onset of gout.

This bring to mind an amusing story about water. A fellow I know could only get motivated to diet if it involved competition. He had two friends who were massively overweight too so it was easy to get a wager going. The plan was to weigh in, nude, each week and whoever lost the most would be paid $10 a pound by the other two.

This sly fellow figured all was fair in love, war and

weight reduction contests. He knew how to win. The evening before the first weigh-in, he started drinking water. He drank glass after glass.

He continued in the morning until his friends arrived. He literally could hear the water sloshing around in his stomach. He had to urinate in the worst way, but he was detemined not to until they had all weighed in.

When the others arrived they stripped down. They didn't notice my friend's discomfort. He even offered them a can of diet soda which they refused. Then, each of the three got on the scale.

One of the others was skeptical. He couldn't believe that my friend weighed as much as the scale read. "You don't have metal weights between your toes?" he asked. But since they were all nude, they could detect nothing fishy.

After they left, my friend quickly made for the bathroom to relieve himself. The next weigh-in was scheduled for the following Friday. As my friend saw it, he could eat as much as he liked and still "win" the bet since he had managed to drink fourteen pounds' worth of water.

The following Friday my friend did, indeed, "win" his bet. But he was just kidding himself.

It's an amusing story, but I hope the point is clear. My friend didn't take off any weight.

Don't kid yourself. If you aren't honest, all your effort will be wasted. Had my friend used his energy for dieting he might have lost the bet but won, by losing pounds. If you want to continue fooling yourself, put this book away and postpone your plans to get thin until you can.

Better to accept yourself as fat than to keep trying and not succeeding, blaming forces other than yourself. A variation of the above trick is frequently used by pregnant women. I recall my first visit to the obstetrician after learning of my pregnancy. Part of the routine during visits was a monthly weigh-in.

Although there has been some difference of opinion about how much weight a woman should gain while she is pregnant, at the time I was carrying my child, getting very heavy was discouraged. An eighteen to twenty pound weight gain was considered ideal.

On that first visit there was another woman in the waiting room with me. Her dress consisted of many different layers of clothing. She seemed to be perspiring due to the weight of her garments.

I asked her if she wasn't uncomfortable dressed that way. "Sure," she replied, "but I want to weigh in heavy this month so that next month, even if I gain weight, I'll still be ahead."

Ahead of what?

I discovered other women who would crash diet the week before their weigh-in with the doctor for the same purpose.

Not only do they deceive themselves, they may be cheating their unborn child. During pregnancy, it's particularly important for women to maintain a balanced diet. That's one time you don't want to be on a reducing plan, unless your physician feels that you are overweight to start out. And then, you must work with him.

If you want to play tricks, use the ones that will *help* you lose weight and not be merely the illusion of accomplishment. By now you have learned many hints that can help you reduce.

In the next chapter we will concentrate on even more "tricks" that can work for you—and make losing weight a winning experience. They *can* make the difference between staying where you are, and getting thinner.

Tricks of the Trade-Off

So you really want to get thin? You want to learn all those little things that make it easy? I remind you again that I didn't promise it would be easy, did I? It is never really easy.

But it *is* possible. It takes preparation, and often it takes a sense of humor.

If you remember that you are always trading one thing off for another more desirable thing you'll get the idea. Trading off some foods and undisciplined eating habits for more positive behavior and a better figure makes the trade worth it.

I will recite a bag full of tricks; some of them I believe will work and others I don't have much faith in. However, I'll give you my opinion as well as that of other people who do think they help. You'll be able to pick and choose from the lot.

Remember walking? How about walking up a flight of

stairs instead of taking the elevator even if you can only make it one floor. Walk down if walking up doesn't appeal to you. It may not be much, but it's something.

If you drop something, retrieve it effectively. By that I mean either with knee bends or leaning straight over from the waist. Turn an accident into an exercise. (Entertainer Rita Moreno uses this as a regular part of her fitness program.)

Once in a while walk to one destination where you would normally take your car. It saves gas and gets you moving.

Keep a picture of yourself in your wallet. A real fat one. If you can't bear the thought of someone discovering it, cut off the head. No one will ever guess it's you. Look at it from time to time, especially when some tempting food is in sight.

Forget about pasting a photo of yourself on the refrigerator or little signs that say things like DON'T BE A DIET DROPOUT. They soon became invisible. If you do want to hang up a picture, choose one where you look great. (This will obviously work only if you have such a photo available!)

Try to eat all your meals in one specific place. This is more difficult than it sounds but if you combine it with the excellent advice to never eat standing up, it's even tougher—and better!

Not eating while standing up immediately eliminates ice cream cones while strolling, pizza from a fast-food counter, hot-dog stands—a giant leap forward.

Apply the rule at home too. The next time you find

yourself nibbling on a potato chip, or even a carrot stick, make sure you sit down at the dining room table.

The point of this is to make eating conscious behavior. If you force yourself to eat only at the table, you must also become aware of the unconscious eating you do. Consciously or unconsciously, it all counts.

Do you know any of the many mothers who turn themselves into human garbage pails? Those are the ones who finish their kids' meals. Half a peanut butter and jelly sandwich here, four French fries there. Then they can't understand how they became fat because they "never eat lunch." They never eat their *own* lunch, that is.

Concentrate on your eating. Eat slowly. *Taste* the food. Don't read while eating. *Never* eat while watching television.

One trick I've used for years is something I used to be somewhat embarrassed about. Until I met other people who do it, too. Moreover, it's recommended by behavior modification experts! Use small plates and utensils. I'll put my food on a little plate and use a small cake fork instead of a large one. That way my smaller portion of food doesn't look lost. If I put two ounces of anything on a large plate just looking at it will make me feel deprived.

If you can manipulate them, use chopsticks. Not only will it slow you down at first, but you'll become accustomed to eating smaller amount of food rather than stuffing your mouth.

Try switching eating hands. If you are right handed, eat with the left, and vice versa.

How about serving yourself exactly one half of the normal portion you usually eat? Then, if you want second helpings, your second portion will actually be the last half of your usual first portion.

If some of these suggestions sound funny, save laughing until you've tried them. You'll find they work. While you're laughing, remember to put down your fork between bites, and swallow before taking more food into your mouth.

I'm sounding more and more like your mother, aren't I?

Except you must retrain yourself out of eating habits that you learned as a child. It's amazing how unaware you are until you start trying to change.

More advice: prepare your plate in the kitchen and put on it the quantity of food you want to eat. Some people suggest that you cook only that amount. This is not always realistic. It's kind of hard to roast six ounces of beef at a time. But it is possible to put that amount on your plate, carry it into the dining room and sit down at the table to eat it.

Wrap and store all leftovers immediately after you have served yourself. Don't make it easy to have a second helping.

Don't put platters of food on the table. If you decide you want more, you'll have to get up and repeat the entire exercise. You may still choose to have that second portion, but you will have made a conscious decision to do so.

Here's another one. Do not eat unless you are hungry. In the early part of this book I told you how efficient my body is just before I find I'm hungry. The world-famous Hindu religious leader, Mahatma Gandhi, said: "An empty stomach is one of the secrets of any creativity."

You may not find your creative juices flowing because of an empty belly, but your gastric juices will start up. It's probably a long time since you've even allowed it to go to half empty. Most of us eat not because we're hungry, but because it's "time to eat." This is one habit we can break.

One of the pleasures of being an adult is that no one tells you to eat. You're the boss. If you don't feel like eating, don't. You will find yourself hungrier for your meals, and you will enjoy them more even while you eat less because the food is truly functioning as fuel.

It could be difficult for people who travel frequently from country to country to follow the advice just offered. Remember that there are great time differences. A friend of mine solved that problem by eating only according to his local time. This sometimes means he gets hungry at three in the morning. But he finds that if he does not do this he constantly throws his body off .

Your problem is not that of a jet traveler. You just want to start recognizing the symptoms of being hungry.

I described how I find myself going right to the kitchen when I arrive home from work. Although I try to keep things available that are good for me to eat, it's even better when I distract myself into some other activity.

How often have you eaten something so quickly you didn't have a chance to think about it? It went down so fast you hardly tasted it. When you learn that it takes the body twenty minutes to "register" the food you've consumed, you can see how impulsive eating is something we very much want to stop.

Before you've reminded yourself you shouldn't, you have already consumed a handful of peanuts, a chocolate brownie, etc. If you can get yourself out of the rooms containing food and give yourself enough time to plan, you'll be on the way to cutting down on these impulses.

How about skipping a meal? Television personality Bill Boggs finds dinner is easiest to eliminate. Go to bed early once a week and poof, no dinner.

You might even skip eating entirely one day a week. Do I hear a gasp? Many of our most fashionable people believe in this as a way to revive the body after an especially full weekend. You may recall I used to fast on Mondays after stuffing myself all weekend long. You don't have to be overfed in order to do this.

I read about one woman who expands on this by spending the entire day in bed. She feels like a little girl playing hooky from her responsibilities, but she loves it. Her magazines and books and telephone are on the bed, and on a table nearby is a large bottle of mineral water. All day long she sips from the bottle.

Of course, this is not practical for those of us who have a houseful of children, dogs, cats and spouses. But we can try to save one portion of each day just for ourselves.

Skipping dinner (or lunch, or breakfast for that matter) or fasting for one day doesn't sound like a punishment when you have it described as above. It should be a mini-respite, one that you will enjoy trying.

Select a time during the day or evening when you usually get the munchies. Make a pact with yourself that today you will not eat them. You needn't commit yourself beyond one day. That's punishment. This is intended to be a positive experience. You will learn that you *can* do it and feel good when you have done it. Just once. It's a contract you are making with yourself. If you want to renegotiate tomorrow, fine. If not, try something else.

In a pamphlet entitled *The Psychology of Dieting*, H. Jon Geis, Ph.D., points out that "can't" nearly always means "won't" or "haven't."

In other words, you are more able to be successful and even to withstand the stress involved in reducing if you discard the concept "I can't."

Dr. Geis says, "It is useful to think in terms of 'I won't' instead of 'I can't' as a way of showing yourself that you *do* have the power to diet successfully if you want to. The word 'can't' implies a 100 per cent prediction with certainty . . ."

If you keep telling yourself "I can't," you probably will be unsuccessful. You are establishing a conclusion before you even start. If you tell yourself "I haven't" that at least leaves open the possibility that you will succeed.

Do you realize that trying your own combination of these hints once, you'll make progress in losing weight and probably never be bored? I believe strongly in varying your routine so you are constantly stimulated in a forward direction. Boredom is a major contribution to overeating. Varying your routine will avoid that trap.

More games: Make it difficult to overeat. If you live alone, keep very little food in the house. If you want food, go out and buy it. Or, take only enough money with you one day to buy a piece of fruit for lunch.

Focus your mind on *trying* to succeed. If your focus is on *trying* rather than on succeeding you reduce the tension and anxiety that can develop when too much importance is placed on success. Don't worry about succeeding. If you follow my advice, winning will take care of itself.

Further, if your aim is to try, you won't be devastated when you occasionally don't live up to your promise.

What's that? Failure? Look, we're human beings. We got fat because we sometimes lose control. You may fall off the wagon occasionally. Later, I'll tell you how to get off a binge. For the moment, I want you to accept yourself, warts and all.

Accepting yourself means also accepting the fact that sometimes it will seem like your plan is falling apart. It's not, really. There are moments when you can try to find out what's really bothering you instead of ignoring your problems by eating.

Overeating will be part of us for a long time; maybe forever. Lots of people still occasionally overeat but manage to stay thin. Because you have been accustomed to being heavy, you might believe that anytime you lose control it means total failure. This is not so. Just as you did not make yourself fat with one isolated moment of overeating, remember too that losing control once in a while is not going to put all the weight back on you.

I can't tell you how many dieters want to throw in the towel because they've had a dessert at dinner. One reason for this reaction is dieters think they are being "good" if they don't have any of the foods they believe make them fat.

By now you know that no food makes you fat. *You* make you fat. Think of the quantity of food you would need to *keep* you fat, and you'll get the idea.

The feeling of deprivation is one which short-circuits many dieters. If you believe that dieting means you are never going to be able to eat your favorite foods you certainly will feel deprived. However, if you *plan* to include them in your diet, you won't feel deprived. *If* you want that dessert, *plan* to eat it occasionally. Look forward to it. You'll undoubtedly enjoy it more than you ever did when you ate it unconsciously. And it won't make you fat. Having fulfilled your desire, you can continue losing.

You may be surprised to discover that once the bugaboo of fear is off "treat" foods, you may not eat them in the quantities you previously did when you were in your uncontrolled state. Now that you don't have to "steal" that treat, a little may go a long way.

Don't forget, when you decide to eat a favorite food, *trade it off against something else.* You can't have it all, but if you enjoy one food more than another, it's worth making the exchange. Most thin people eat this way. For them it's automatic.

Deprivation is a negative force; reducing is a positive

one. *When you have reduced you will feel good about yourself.* Every step you take to lose pounds should make you feel that you are taking a positive action. The feeling will sustain your effort and will propel you forward.

Control can be a positive force in your life. Look upon controlled eating as beneficial. If you don't agree with me, think about the uncontrolled eating you have done and recall how unhappy you were about it and about its result.

If you think about spending the rest of your life on a diet, the thought will depress you. But if you think of gaining control of your eating and, thus, your life, you can look forward to great and good feelings with possible serendipity rewards.

Compulsive eating and belly-filling bingeing are uncontrolled. I've never met anyone who claims to really enjoy the experience. The morning after—even the hour after—is often miserable. You are filled with self-recrimination and an abiding sense of failure.

Let's continue to examine the positives.

Do you weigh yourself too often? There are many theories about weighing. I have tested all of them from weighing myself every day to weighing myself everytime I got to the bathroom, to weighing myself once a week.

Want to know something? It doesn't matter. When we thin out, the evidence will be there, whether or not we see a number recorded in front of our eyes. People go nutty about scales and their messages.

When I subscribe to the daily weigh-in regime, I get on the scale at the same time each day, completely stripped, after going to the bathroom.

Weight is relative and scales vary. Don't panic when you step on someone else's scale and see a different number than you saw on your own.

I'm very attached to my scale. It's like an old friend. I consider it "correct," because I weigh myself only on my own scale. The fact is, it doesn't matter if my scale is "right" or "wrong" since it is the only guide I use.

Discover what's best for you and keep in mind that your weight will fluctuate, not only weekly and daily, but within the day, too. (After eating, I can "weigh" four pounds more!)

Whether or not you weigh yourself, if you are eating according to your food plan, you are winning. The number on the scale is not the point. Getting thin is.

You're Going to Be Eating

You are going to be eating, so let's discuss rather than avoid talk about food. Start with your own special favorites. Some people enjoy cottage cheese and grapefruit while others cringe at the sight of either one of them.

I can eat chicken every day. If you can too, prepare a different (or the same, if you wish) chicken meal for every day of the week. It may bore someone else, but for you it's perfect, and nutritious. Next week, switch to a different food. For me, steak is another favorite, although higher priced. If I don't include your favorites, substitute them.

If you are lucky enough and rich enough to be a Jacqueline Onassis you can prepare a simple 500 calorie meal with a baked potato topped off with a generous dollop of Beluga caviar.

Often, when I decide to get purposeful to knock off

the few pounds that have crept up on me, I limit my food to the protein variety. If you're lucky enough to have a fat bankroll this can be a pleasurable way to take off the weight.

If you can afford shrimp, lobster, caviar, steak (lean cuts, please) you'll see what I mean. Of course, fish (not so cheap anymore, either), chicken, tuna fish, cottage cheese, and eggs are also available, so don't count high protein out if you're on a budget.

Although I don't recommend fad diets, sometimes the one-sided eating approach can be effective. Anything that is going to help you lose weight is acceptable, provided it is for a short time and not totally outlandish.

When I separated from my husband and decided to drop some weight, I ate just about the same thing every day. It was either a steak and salad or a large hamburger and salad, depending on my budget.

The effectiveness of this menu was largely due to its monotony. Although I've warned you that boredom and deprivation can lead to going off your diet, in this case, it was my choice, not a program forced on me. *Choice* is the important difference.

This will only work for those of you for whom varying your menu leads to an over-concentration about food. If you are going to think all day about how you might create a masterpiece out of 350 calories, I don't know if you are learning to change your focus away from food to other interests.

Think about whether eating the same, albeit nutritious, menu for one week straight will bore the life out of you and make you crave hot fudge sundaes. If your answer is yes, go for variety. However, if eating the same food eliminates thinking about and worrying over what you'll have for dinner, this may be an effective approach.

Don't make it absurd—don't eat only strawberries and pickled herring. Make sure you select food that will nourish your body. You can pick foods you genuinely like. Making your *own* choices makes for enjoyment; when someone *else* decides for you it can lead to feeling deprived. *Your involvement is what makes the critical difference.*

By planning in advance that you will eat an eight ounce hamburger and a green salad with oil and vinegar, you won't hurt yourself one bit. And, if you like, toss in a glass of red wine. Light a candle, put on the stereo and have a pleasant time.

As you might be able to tell, I very enthusiastically endorse this approach. If you want variety, do it on a change-the-menu-each-week basis.

Keep foremost in mind that your goal is to lose weight, not to plan menus.

When I was a youngster attending junior high school, I ate cream cheese and jelly sandwiches every schoolday for one solid year. I guess I was cut out for this lifestyle. I can still taste those sandwiches and enjoy their memory. (By the way, I haven't had a cream cheese and jelly sandwich since then!)

If you care to, figure out a menu that contains the precise number of calories you want to consume daily.

Write it down.

Make it a simple one.

Eat that same menu for one week.

Many dieters respond well to the above since it takes the day-to-day or meal-to-meal planning out of their hands.

Taking the surprise element out of food is helpful when you want to lose weight. Part of this approach is to make food seem less important in the full scope of your life. In time, when you have won the battle against your bulges, you can be more flexible. But at the beginning it's safer to know in advance what's going down.

It may turn you into a person who starts looking at the rest of the world instead of only restaurants, food articles, and the like. You will find yourself not thinking about dinner and maybe planning instead what film to see, or what book you are going to read.

Dining is an incredibly social activity. Thus, when behavior modification specialists tell us to make eating an isolated experience they're asking a great deal.

Just as I don't think it is a solution to go to a spa and lose weight under controlled conditions, I also concede that making eating a "pure" experience may not work for you. So, if you *must* watch TV or read a newspaper while eating—make sure your quantity controls are firmly set first.

This reminds me of a friend whose excuse for not dieting is that he has to go to his villa on the island of Jamaica to isolate himself, if he is to diet. But what happens when he comes out of isolation?

The sooner you learn to lose weight right in the middle of the real world, the sooner you're going to win the war. Needing to be isolated is only another cop out.

When I was a Weight Watcher—at my fattest—I managed to lose weight, although, as I mentioned, it was in the middle of the Thanksgiving and Christmas holiday season.

If you are motivated it doesn't matter where you are. You can be sitting in a pool of Swiss butter almond ice cream surrounded by mounds of Almond Joy candy bars, platters of hot pizza and mountains of Black Forest chocolate cake and they will all seem like chunks of dead wood to you.

I concede that it's practically unpatriotic to not socialize with people unless there is food available. Think about the last time you were invited out to a friend's home. Did you sit and enjoy each other's company without nibbling? At what hour was coffee and cake served? Or was the event a party where the onset of the food platters seemed to be the high point of the evening?

It would probably start a small revolution to suggest to people that they can relate without watching each other chew. Care to join me in a peaceful revolution?

Relax. You don't have to struggle to change the world. All you need change is yourself. You are going to learn how to live with food and still lose weight.

If you find you need support on a one-to-one basis I highly recommend consulting a behavior modification specialist. It's becoming more popular for physicians to work together with such experts since these are the people who are trained in nutrition and who can help tailor a reducing regime to your particular needs.

Where most diets fail is that they don't take you further than the weight loss. However, if your weight reduction program is designed with foods that you can continue eating after the weight is off, you're headed for the winner's circle.

Behavior modification is important enough to merit a separate chapter. However before we talk more about modifying your behavior, let's do more plain talking about food.

I'm deliberately not advocating that you eat specific foods or recommending one reducing approach over another because I want you to be able to make decisions for yourself.

I keep stressing that no one food or diet program will work for everyone. Your needs and desires are probably different from mine, so it's not fair for me to tell you that every day you will eat certain foods and then you'll be thin.

Instead, I have encouraged you to select those foods you enjoy eating. If you include them in your reducing program, you will lose weight without sacrificing pleasurable eating.

Most important of all, the foods you choose will be foods that you'll be able to continue to eat after you lose the weight.

This is not merely a diet, it's a new way of life.

More Talk About Food

Occasionally I'll read through a supposed "diet" food recipe for cheesecake or the like. There are so many substitutes for ingredients that would make you fat that you end up with an imitation that would seem more at home in a chemistry laboratory than a kitchen.

My philosophy is that there are no forbidden foods. Only forbidden ways to eat them. With that in mind, I suggest you have cheescake if you want it. Good cheese-cake is too delicious to mess around with substitutes. If you think you ought not eat it, wait until you feel you can.

Good things are worth waiting for. The fake is just that: fake.

And while you're at it, don't fool yourself about "natural" foods. Everyone is turned on these days when they see a package labeled "natural." Dr. Scrimshaw, whom I quoted earlier, says the notion that such foods are safe is "a total myth."

He adds, "A surprisingly high percentage of the food we eat and think of as natural has toxic substances that wouldn't pass the rat tests required of all additives. A list of these substances includes hemaglutins in beans, cyanogenic glycosides in almonds and lima beans, pressor amines in bananas, pineapples, lemons, tomatoes, sauerkraut juice, Stilton and Camembert cheeses and even natural radioactivity in some drinking water."

Whatever these things are, I don't want them in my body!

I'm not asking you to toss in the towel completely on "natural" foods, but don't be fooled into thinking they are going to save you or the rest of the world.

There are now many "natural" and "health food" stores. Have you ever wondered how natural some of them are? Not far from my home there is one such shop. You can find natural vitamins, natural cookies, sprouts and so forth. Even natural and organically grown fresh vegetables. And not surprisingly, these foods frequently cost a lot more than "unnatural" ones.

A neighbor of mine shopped in this store often. She developed a personal friendship with the woman who owned the shop. One morning when my neighbor was browsing in the shop, the owner took my friend aside. Evidencing some discomfort, she advised my neighbor not to buy the carrots. When asked why, the natural health food store owner revealed that they were purchased at the local supermarket—not from an organic farm.

I suppose she felt guilty that day and decided to save my friend the considerable difference it would have cost since the carrots were marked up to the suitable "natural" price.

I do not mean to suggest that all, or even many of these shops are run this way. However, you might be surprised at how many perfectly acceptable products you can find right in your supermarket.

(And I'll never forget the anger on the face of natural health foods advocate Simon Gould when he related the experience of entering an organically grown vegetable shop in which he was a shareholder only to come upon a clerk spraying the fruits and vegetables with an insecticide.)

Some dieters decide that becoming vegetarian is going to solve all their weight problems, and, at the same time, they'll be "healthier." While it is certainly true that you can get all the nutrition you need through a vegetarian diet (proteins can be derived from many foods other than animal flesh—milk, cheese, whole grains, etc.) don't think that you will become thin automatically. There are plenty of overweight vegetarians. Some of them eat their way through huge masses of nuts, grains, etc., and these can put on pounds.

Vegetarianism is fine, if it's comfortable for you. I find myself eating less beef and other red meats, partly because they contain more calories and partly because they are frequently the most expensive items you can buy. However, I'm not committed to any -ism when it comes to food.

Keep in mind the critical point I've tried to make again and again. For your food program to be effective it must be one that you'll be satisfied living with for years to come. If you think vegetarianism fits that bill, try it.

Vegetarian cooks frequently are very creative since they need to invent interesting ways to prepare the foods they buy. I believe one reason many of us are "meat and potatoes people" is because it's somehow simpler to grill a steak or chop. It takes some flair to make eggplant fascinating.

There are many foods that can be helpful to you in reducing. You'll have to decide which of the ones I mention are for you and substitute others of equal caloric value for those that don't appeal to you.

At this stage in your dieting career (since many of us have made it just that) you probably can judge calories fairly well. I don't have to tell you that celery has fewer calories than corn.

Ideally, I'd like you to stop counting calories. Work with foods that you know in advance are not fattening. That way you don't have to spend your energy figuring how much roast pork and applesauce you can fit into 200 calories!

I find that with a food that is low in calories, I don't need to know how much of it I can eat. I just eat. It always works.

Carryl Atton,* the behavior modification specialist I mentioned earlier, made a suggestion worth repeating. It's simple and effective:

---

* Carryl Atton is located at 7 Park Avenue in Manhattan (New York, N.Y. 10017). Her telephone number is (212) 684 3672.

Always have available in your refrigerator a small bowl of carrot sticks and celery (or radishes, sliced cabbage, cucumber, etc.). They must be fresh and appetizing to the eye and instantly visible. That means you cover the dish lightly with plastic wrap (not aluminum foil, which would make it invisible).

In a day or two discard any shriveled up leftovers. Sure, this may cost a few cents, but these vegetables are much cheaper than most junk foods. You are making an investment in a new figure. You are worth it.

A sociologist from Hofstra University on Long Island, New York, tells us that Americans alone spend $1,400,-000,000 a year trying to lose weight. *A billion four hundred million!* This includes "a billion dollars on diet food, books and literature and $220 million a year at health spas and weight-reducing salons."

If you consider all that money, tossing out old vegetables will seem a mere drop in the expense bucket.

Along with the veggies keep a similar dish with bite-size pieces of chicken. (Just in case you didn't already know this, remove the skin, even if you love it.)

When you come home hungry and hit the refrigerator, the first thing you should see are these two dishes. I'm not about to promise that you will always eat these "good" foods. But even if you turn to them fifty percent of the time, you are halfway there.

You may surprise yourself and even learn to like and yes, even prefer, these to other, more fattening snacks. Crunchy foods satisfy an essential urge to chew. It doesn't have to be pretzels; carrots fill the need equally.

If you have the kind of job that allows it, take similar nibbles to work with you. These days no one will think you are weird for toting your own food around. On the contrary, in the world of jet set society, hardly anybody eats anything anymore.

People are sipping mineral waters instead of martinis at business lunches and the most chic people rarely, if ever, allow themselves the luxury of eating the bread that is placed on the plate next to their left. The waiter puts the bread down, you smile, and he knows he'll be taking it away, untouched later.

Professional lunchers rarely have dessert. Take my word for it, we are headed for the non-lunch lunch.

You carry your plastic bag or container of raw cauliflower and you'll be the envy of your peers who'll be having indigestion over greasy hamburgers.

If you are still not convinced that you can comfortably carry this off, just bear in mind that it's all in your style. If you act like you are supposed to be behaving in a certain way, no one ever questions you. They admire you.

The actress Carol Channing, best known for her portrayal of Dolly Levi in the Broadway musical, *Hello Dolly*, always carries her own food wherever she goes. And that includes restaurants. No one ever questions her when she produces her little package.

To repeat: It's all in your style. So have some flair when you whip out your baggie of goodies.

Let's talk salt.

Everyone knows that the rule is to reduce salt intake on a diet. But are you aware of the reason for the rule? Salt causes your body to retain water. Even if you know that water isn't real weight, when you feel bloated, you feel bloated. If you feel fat you may feel depressed. And, if you feel depressed . . . you may start eating. So, even though you know that the first weight you lose when you start a new diet is water, it's still uplifting to know that something is coming off.

Some people swear that salt has absolutely no effect on their fluid retention, while others blow up. If possible, cut down on salt. If you can't live without corned beef, eat it. But trade it off against the salted peanuts.

In addition to salt, fats and sweets can also cause edema.

I recently stopped salting my food. Not because of fluid retention but because my doctor told me I have a tendency towards high blood pressure. Since I already described my family history in morbid detail, you'll recall that all of them had high blood pressure.

I've cut down on salt. If food is presalted, I don't add any. You'd be amazed at how many people salt their food automatically before they even taste it.

Taste first before adding salt. If you think the food needs it, add it, sparingly. You may discover new food tastes that you were masking with the salt.

How about chewing gum? There are different opinions about chewing gum and I agree with all of them. I'll explain. Some say chewing gum replaces the need to eat, if only temporarily. Others believe that chewing will start you salivating and will turn on your appetite. Both can be true.

Sometimes not having anything in your mouth will stall your urge to eat because your appetite button hasn't been switched on. But there are other moments when you just have to have it. When that happens find a brand of chewing gum that has few calories (lots of these are available) and one that keeps its flavor and softness.

You might think I'm carrying on a bit much about chewing gum. However, often these "little" things make a big difference between success and failure. If you are chewing gum that gets hard fast and loses its flavor quickly, you are going to dispose of it and start another piece. And those few calories can add up.

Even with sugarless chewing gum, moderation, as the ancient Greeks said, is the best policy. I currently prefer Carefree peppermint gum. It's a generous stick, and fulfills both requirements for me.

While we're at it, let's talk about low calorie candies. There are some that contain three or four calories. With candy, I feel pretty much the same as with other pretend foods. One piece of candy isn't going to make you fat; many pieces do. And, with low calorie candy, if you don't watch your intake, you may discover you have consumed as much or more than you might have if you had indulged in one piece of the real McCoy.

Is having one piece of candy going to turn you into the Candy Monster who devours everything in sight? If you *honestly* think you can manage to have one piece, eat it. You may find yourself more satisfied that way.

And, that sense of satisfaction can propel you forw:
As we well know, the feeling of deprivation does not make good diet sense.

If you recall, I used candy as a diet trick, eating a piece before meals. It worked for me. But since you promised to be realistic about losing weight, you'll have to be realistic about this too. If you think you cannot eat just one piece of candy, don't have any at all, not even the low calorie type. Maybe the calories won't be hurting you, but if sweetness turns on your hungries, whether it's low or high in calories, it is better to pass it by.

As dieters, we recognize the negative effect of sugar on our bodies. There are scientists who insist that sugar is not a food at all and if it was to be introduced today as a new additive, the Food and Drug Administration would ban it as unfit for human consumption.

Sugar can be addictive. It puts your body chemistry into a sudden high, and then there is an equally sudden low which creates an irrational desire for more sugar. There is also increasing evidence that sugar may be a contributing factor in high blood pressure. An Associated Press story described the results of research at Louisiana State University involving monkeys. It was found "that monkeys on a diet of high salt and sugar experienced a rise in blood pressure exceeding that of monkeys fed only a high salt diet."

They are not yet saying that humans will react exactly the way monkeys do, but the thrust of the evidence points accusingly against sugar.

You may grumble from time to time because you have to make decisions about eating or not eating certain foods at certain times. Why haven't I simply outlined a day-by-day plan for you to follow? Most other diet books do that. But you have tried those and once the diet is ended, your climb up the scales begins again. I have *you* selecting your own food instead of relying on formula diets, so that from the beginning you are in charge of your own behavior.

Let's examine this attitude of responsibility in another part of your life for a moment. Unless you are home-bound because of illness, you probably select your own clothing when you go shopping. Sure, you may ask your spouse or friends for their opinion, but the final decision is yours. It probably wouldn't occur to you to hand over to someone else the job of choosing your wardrobe. It should make the same good sense to select your own foods.

When we began we agreed that you were going to take charge of your life. If you continue to let Dr. Atkins or Dr. Stillman or anyone else dictate what you eat, you'll never grow up. You don't need that crutch. You can be in control.

There's no better feeling for a person who has struggled for years with weight than the satisfaction of losing it and keeping it off.

We know that meat is high not only in calories, but in fat as well. Do you like fish? Then eat lots of it.

Fish is so low in calories that almost anything you do in preparing fish can't add up to the calories you consume in a big steak. Nine ounces of sirloin steak contains 750 calories. Nine ounces of haddock, breaded and fried, contains 420 calories. And that includes the fat for frying it!

I'm not suggesting that you deep fry the fish or use heavy breading in its preparation. However, since it is lower in calories to begin with, you can be more relaxed.

There is another reason to learn how to judge calories without actually getting bogged down in counting them. People start hunting for calorie charts that give slightly better counts. If you search, you *can* find calorie charts where one food may be listed as having fewer calories than on another chart.

Who are you foolin'?

If you want to believe that because a bran muffin is listed in one chart as having 105 calories, every bran muffin has the same count, you're back to playing kiddie games with yourself.

It's better to recognize that certain types of foods are basically higher in calories than others. If you have a question about a food, don't eat it. If you have to ask yourself if that bran muffin you are about to eat is of the 105 calorie variety, chances are excellent that you already know it's not. Leave half of it. Okay, leave the smaller half, but leave something.

As I suggested, if you concentrate on foods that are "good" for you, you won't have to be busy counting calories. However, if you feel you just must have a sirloin steak, go ahead, but follow the firm rule about trading it off for something else.

If you are accustomed to having a baked potato with

your steak, kill that reflex habit that has you adding butter and sour cream without thinking about it. No butter and sour cream!

For years I have cut my baked potato in half and dug out the meat. I give that to my daughter, Jenny. I devour the delicious (and nutritious) crispy skin. (Sometimes I think I was a pioneer. Today it is not uncommon to find potato skins on restaurant menus.)

Incidentally, if you want the skins on baked potatoes to be crisp, don't wrap them in aluminum foil. Even if it looks pretty, it prevents the skin from crisping.

Let's talk about pasta. No food is forbidden if you handle it intelligently. For many years I swore off all pasta. I promised myself I would eat it only in Italy. (That can be darned effective. Especially if you travel only occasionally, and even less frequently to Italy!)

Now that I control my food most of the time (rather than allowing it to control me), I occasionally do indulge myself with a spaghetti dish. Weight Watchers now include pasta in their food plan. I was first!

The problem with pasta, or other foods that you are used to really chowing down, is that you have to know when it's stop time. I've said that I control food and not the other way round, but I'm also realistic. There are devious foods lurking everywhere that want to take the command position away from me. Being realistic about pasta is knowing I find it hard to limit the quantity I eat.

I ask myself if I will be able to eat only a little. The two-thirds of a cup of cooked pasta recommended by Weight Watchers is not an enormous portion. Cutting the long strands of spaghetti into pieces so tiny that you turn that two-thirds of a cup into quite a generous serving is self-defeating.

If you catch yourself cheating on the measuring, you're on dangerous ground. Beware of quicksand and quagmires. Remind yourself that when you cheat, you are the victim. Put the pasta away until you are absolutely certain that a little will be enough.

If any food seems too challenging when you are trying to lose weight, don't add to your problems.

One approach to losing weight that works for me is a rule I try to stick to: *IF YOU DON'T KNOW WHAT'S IN IT, DON'T EAT IT!*

Thus, if you eat pasta at a restaurant with marinara sauce, etc., you can never be certain of the ingredients. If you make it in your home you have control.

I shy away from Chinese food, which I adore, for much the same reason. Most Americans have been brainwashed into believing that if you eat Chinese food you will be "hungry again in an hour."

Whoever said that hasn't observed what I order in a Chinese restaurant. Platter after platter is brought to the table offering not merely tempting vegetable dishes, but succulent pork and duck and beef. Gone is the Chinese restaurant style of the 1930s where Chinese food consisted of a little meat sprinkled on a pile of sometimes unidentifiable vegetables.

Chinese cuisine is considered one of the two great cuisines of the world, and you can eat too much of it just as you can of any other food.

I stay away from Chinese food because often the

recipes are so complex that I just don't know what ingredients go into its preparation. Using my motto as a guide, I don't know what's in it, so it's not part of my regular food program.

I don't feel that I'm punishing myself. When I do decide to have Chinese food, it's a genuine treat. And when I eat it, I enjoy it without any thought of what it's doing to my figure. I trade off the Chinese food that I have that day by cutting down the next day. Or, by cutting down on other foods that same day.

Unless you understand that you cannot eat the Chinese food *and* all the rest of the food you usually do, you'll stay fat forever. On the other hand, just as soon as you begin to balance your food, you're on the way towards becoming thin *and* learning to be flexible about food.

Am I convincing you that *you* supply all the magic necessary to get thin? Believe me, your magic is greater than the promises and schemes of "experts" who haven't been through the struggle themselves. I've not only been there, but I've managed to win. I stay thin. I feel good. I look good. And I eat all the kinds of foods that I thoroughly enjoy.

Isn't mine a lovely situation to be in?

There's room for you right beside me. You can do it too. You can experience how great it feels to have people look at you with the same envy that you used to have for thinnies. You'll appreciate and enjoy it as I do.

Never for one minute do I take my thinness for granted. Every day I wake up pleased with the job I've accomplished. I want you to share this terrific feeling.

Before I had full confidence in my ability to live without certain foods, I used to buy "diet" things. One such item was "diet" jam or jelly, made with low-calorie sweetener. This is much like the cheesecake I mentioned before. Yucch. It does not taste like "real" jelly or jam. The useful purpose it may serve is to turn you off using jams altogether.

We are so trusting, so unaccustomed to investigating. Imagine how surprised I was to read the ingredients label on a jar of the real thing. This label included the caloric value of one tablespoon's worth of jam. I discovered that it was well within reasonable limits for food that I could include in my eating program.

In other words, I didn't *have* to use the substitute. We always assume that certain foods are "fattening" and so reach for the lo-cal variety. Now that many foods are being labeled so that you can know their precise ingredients and caloric content, you'll find there are foods you can have in your diet that you used to exclude.

You will save money (since the lo-cal versions are invariably more expensive), enjoy the taste of real food, and still continue to reduce.

Lately, I have seen jams on sale that, instead of using artificial sweetener, whose taste many people dislike, have reduced sugar content. Apparently there is a demand for products that are "real" and yet less sweet than traditional.

I don't eat bread. But bread may be important to you.

If so, it's not difficult to cut in half the amount of bread you usually eat. Use one slice instead of two. They do this in Scandinavia and call it smorrebrod. You can, if you wish, put the same total contents on one-half the portion of bread.

I'm always amazed at how some behavior which we think is universal may only be a habit we've acquired. Since I use bread so infrequently at home, I've observed that Jenny is not keen on sandwiches. There are school lunches which do not use bread.

Jenny prefers soups, pieces of cheese, etc. Her best friend, Elissa, rarely eats a traditional sandwich. From her school chums who are Japanese she learned about what she calls "Japanese" sandwiches. Whether they're authentic or not, I'll leave to you to check. But Elissa uses a leaf of Iceberg lettuce instead of bread. In the lettuce leaf she places a bit of meat, or chicken, or whatever, and then rolls it up.

Should you be skeptical, let me assure you that these are tricks that people use, *and they work*. Consider anything that may work for you. Don't worry about looking foolish. Keep your get-thin goal clearly in sight.

Each time you set a plate of food before you, decide in your mind to leave something on it. Even a carrot. It's a symbol of self discipline to not consume everything in sight.

We've talked about the myth called "will power." There is another, more persistent instinct. You can use it to full advantage. I call it "want power." You want one thing more than you want another. In this instance you want to be thin more than you want to stay fat.

Once you've got a bellyful of "want power" your problem is licked. Remember this each time you are in a temptation situation. Eventually, it will become part of you.

FIVE RULES TO LIVEN UP
YOUR LIGHTENING UP

1. Small portions of many foods.
2. Keep refrigerated snacks of fresh vegetables.
3. Better a small portion of "real" food than an abundance of artificial "diet" feed.
4. Give gifts of the things you love to eat to other people. Treat them to restaurant desserts and feel proud of yourself as you watch them eat it.
5. Pick one food that makes you fat and avoid it for seven days. Vary this from week to week.

Change
Is the Magic Word

Change. That's what it's all about, isn't it? Trade offs.
Awareness. Choices.

SUCCESS IS YOURS FOR THE TAKING
IF YOU TRULY WANT IT

I have been telling you in plain talk that the answers
are within you. It seems easier to believe that outside
influences make you fat. That way you can wrap yourself up in your overweight, throw up your hands in
frustration and feel sorry for yourself.

When you believe others make you fat you are easy
prey for the next crazy diet to come along. So if that's
the attitude you are comfortable with, put this book
aside until you are ready for change.

Ah, but you have come this far with me, so I must be
getting through to you. Stay with me and you will end
up like me—thin.

Have you matured enough to accept reality? Are you

now ready to admit that you simply cannot lose weight eating jelly beans for one week and expect to keep it off?

Are you ready to change your eating attitudes?

Now you know you needn't panic because you think you won't ever bite into a hero sandwich again. Now you know that you'll be able to eat anything you want.

I am a thin person. I eat fantastically well. And I'm not talking about boring, "diet" food. By now you know there is no food that is forbidden: you can eat anything if you know how to handle it.

Isn't it more than just a little fascinating that "dieting" has come to mean going without food? Diet isn't a bad word; it's a word whose definitions we tend to forget. We forget that one definition is simply "a manner of living as regards food." Nothing about fat or thin.

Another definition of diet is "to improve the physical condition." Nothing there about fat or thin, either. (But you know and I know that if we are thin our physical condition is improved.)

It's not crazy to have you ask yourself again at this point, "Do I really want to be thin?"

If the answer is "Yes"—then what are you waiting for?

Think about the question. To get thin and stay that way you must make an agreement with yourself that you are willing to live with.

Are you ready?

Before this book, you might have been concerned about having to give up foods you love. I belong to gourmet groups where I dine on sumptuous wines and exotic foods. I'm thinner now than I ever dreamed I could be, and yet I once worried about giving up my security blanket foods, also.

You will be making decisions about what you are going to eat. *You* may choose foods that appeal most to *you*.

You've learned about tradeoffs. We trade things off against other things every day of our lives.

If you want to go to a film tomorrow night, you don't need me to tell you that you can't attend the ballet at the same time. Translate this to food.

When I was a child, a secret pleasure was one shared with my good friend, Anne. Once in a while we played hooky from school and went to Anne's house, because her mother worked. We had a ritual that never varied.

She always had My-T-Fine chocolate pudding in the pantry. We'd cook up a pot of chocolate pudding and eat it, hot. Right from the pot. We devoured it with no worry about weight or pimples, both of which appeared on our bodies quickly enough.

I think fondly of those days and the My-T-Fine chocolate pudding. If I want chocolate pudding today, I'll have it. If I want to eat the whole portion right out of the pot, I'll do that too. And if I choose to, I'll enjoy it and not feel guilty about it.

BUT—of course there is a "but"—if I choose to eat the chocolate pudding, I am fully willing to trade it off against other foods I might be eating. I cannot have the chocolate pudding *and* my chocolate chip cookie and tea in the evening. I cannot have it *and* eat a sirloin steak and baked potato for dinner. I cannot have that pudding *and* still eat my bran muffin and jam in the morning.

Do I feel deprived? Not at all. Because *if* I want the pudding, I decide I want it more than the other foods. Sometimes I feel it's worth it. Other times I decide it isn't.

I'm dwelling on this because once you accept and embrace it emotionally, your eating life will become a rational one and having been needlessly overweight will come to seem tragic-silly to you.

The most effective change is for you to create your own individual eating plan, structured for your needs.

Since we have explored the positives and negatives of many popular diets, let's explore in depth just how a person trained as a behavior modification expert works. There's some variation, of course, but if a one-to-one relationship is for you, this is pretty much what you can expect.

When my friend Michael went to Carryl Atton for help, he had tried everything. I mean *everything:* Atkins, Stillman, shots in the backside, liquid protein, pills to curb your appetite, pills that promised to change your metabolism within three weeks. Invariably he had lost weight. And invariably he always put it right back on. He often added a pound or two to reach a new high.

He was desperate. Every magic or crash diet had failed. He'd spent thousands of dollars trying to stay thin and it never worked.

He had the problems universal among heavy people. For one thing, although he had been considerably obese for more than twenty years, he never forgot that he had been a thin boy. He was convinced that any day that thin boy would emerge from his fat body. Fat was only a temporary state for him.

This attitude is not detrimental in itself. As a matter of fact, it is an asset. It's positive thinking.

On the other hand, he found it difficult to admit he had a severe problem about dieting. He could point to all the times he had lost weight as proof that it wasn't so.

He had a tremendous ego. It takes superhuman courage for a person who is capable in all other aspects of his life to confess that he has a problem that is out of control.

How many people do you know (maybe even yourself) who keep saying, "Any time I want to, I'll get thin." "Nobody has to help me." "I can do it." Even when he tried Weight Watchers he was convinced that he was different from all those fat people.

What is it about being fat that is such an emotional issue? If your car has a flat tire you don't think it's a personal weakness to have somebody else change it. On the contrary, you're relieved. Admitting you need help to lose weight needn't be any different.

It's no different than alcoholism or drug addiction. Overeating is *your* form of alcoholism, and the first step to the control of alcoholism is admitting you need help.

Admitting he had a problem that he couldn't solve himself was the big step for my friend. Once he admitted to the problem the next step was realizing that *he* was the one preventing a return to his image of the thin boy.

Reality hurt his feelings, but he finally, reluctantly, admitted that being fat was his own doing. Getting him to consult Carryl Atton was not easy. He doubted that anyone could help him get thin; however, he agreed to try.

That was the second step. First he admitted he had a problem and then he was willing to consider that he needed outside help. Personal diet counselling is particularly effective for people like my friend Michael because it is tailor-made for people who respond best to individualized attention.

What is an expert in behavior modification?

A behavior modification counselor is a person who may be trained in nutrition, may or may not be a physician; but she or he is there for you and for you alone. If you question their sincerity, believe that there are easier ways to earn a living than trying to help frustrated overweight people reduce.

Carryl Atton was a compulsive eater herself and had once been extremely obese. When my friend met her she was still plump, although she has become quite slim now. Her personal involvement with weight as well as her training in nutrition showed that she could readily understand the problems of obesity.

You don't have to be fat to know how to reduce, but it can help. Unlike other parts of our lives, if you've been fat, your firsthand experience gives you more understanding of the problems. I was there so I can share your anguish. So could Carryl Atton.

Her approach stresses eating awareness. She doesn't

find it necessary to dig deep into your past to find out why you eat; your present eating patterns are more important. Otherwise, you can spend many months rationalizing about how you were forced to eat as an infant, or forced not to eat, etc., instead of using that time and energy to get thin.

The task is to help you develop certain eating patterns while breaking others, without feeling deprived. You find yourself getting in touch not only with your food needs, but with yourself.

Since no two people are alike, no two programs will be.

When my friend visited her she surprised him by not telling him what he should eat. Rather, she discussed the foods he found enjoyable and encouraged him to continue eating those that were beneficial.

Essentially, you plan your program with her. She shies away from the word "diet." Like many in her field, she encourages keeping a food diary. Through her guidance and your own analysis you will discover those foods that turn on allergic reactions in your body, or which may trigger uncontrolled eating. Obviously, they should be avoided.

A little goes a long way, and my friend left her office, which, by the way, is in her home, very much impressed. Here was a person who neither disapproved nor approved of his fatness. Being fat did not make him a bad person, needing scolding. Being fat was viewed as a problem to be solved.

The second visit was devoted to suggestions on how to

eat. We've discussed many of them: such as putting down the fork between bites, really tasting each food and making eating a pleasurable and total experience. My friend was counseled to close his eyes during a meal in order to feel the taste and textures virtually "explode" with flavor. Try it and see how effective this is.

A behavior modification counselor is not going to be judgmental or people will not return. Slowly, a relationship grew between them until my friend trusted and believed she had his best interests in mind.

She encouraged contact and my friend found himself calling her often during the week, never worrying about disturbing her. She assured him that she was there to buoy his efforts.

Of course, he eventually learned a great deal about eating and was soon on the road to losing weight.

You can change your behavior without a counselor to help. I did it. But if I was losing weight today I'd certainly welcome having a supportive and knowledgable person backing me up.

Think of the times you desperately wanted someone to talk to who would understand. Times when your spouse or best friend just wasn't there. Or worse, was the one who kept you fat!

However you go about modifying your eating behavior is up to you. The group approach of Weight Watchers is supportive. Even more so is Overeaters Anonymous which employs a sponsorship relationship where you have someone assigned to you. That person is a buddy who gets involved with your food problems.

If I hear someone out there saying they can't afford

it, don't forget all the millions of dollars spent each year on diet-related foods. How many of *your* dollars are included in that amount?

Maybe the answer is you can't *not* afford it.

Whether you try a group approach, do it alone, or see a behavior modification expert, this is the time in your life when you have decided that you are never going to go on another diet.

I hope that you've made many promises to yourself in the course of reading this book. Have you promised yourself to be realistic about how much weight you feel you should lose? Are you ready to run your last and most successful race toward *permanent* thinness?

Then let's move up to the starting line.

How to Break a Binge

I'm not predicting you will binge. You may not. However, having been in your place, I know I sometimes do go off the deep end. Even now. If I expected perfect control from myself all the time, those moments I do fall would wipe me out. But remember, we are not always able to be totally in charge.

In the past, if you were average, you went on a diet and stayed on it for two or three or even four days, at which time you got tired or bored and you cheated. Then you felt guilty and discouraged and you were off and running to recover the lost pounds. That's past. We're striking both "guilt" and "discouragement" from our diet vocabulary.

As a realistic dieter, learn to accept yourself as a person who sometimes will eat foods you would prefer not to eat; you occasionally will eat more food than you wish you had; and you will maybe have a binge or two, or three.

I do not mean you should plan to binge. You won't have to! However, if you are aware that it may happen, you will be better able to regain control of yourself and not lose too much ground. As a matter of fact, you may not lose any ground at all.

Here's how it may happen and how you might handle yourself. Your boss has told you he's passing you over this raise period. You come home expecting comfort from your wife and she's not there. There's a note telling you the twins need braces which will cost thousands of unexpected dollars and she's taken them to the orthodontist. She adds the information that she may be late, so please feed the dog and yourself.

What's a man to do? It would be nice to think everyone can handle bad news by saying, "Golly, that's too bad, I'm going to sit down and have a few carrots."

Reality is such that you probably will start "soothing" all your wounds by feeding yourself. Food, as we know, was the original pacifier, as it came from your mother's bosom, or from the bottle. Unfortunately, most people are only made more miserable when they binge. So we want to know how to stop it.

If you expect it to happen once in a while you will be able to abbreviate the duration of your binges. You will be able to look at yourself and say, "I'm doing it again!"

Whatever you do, *don't hate yourself!* Don't feel that this symptom of mortality means that you're "bad" or "a weakling."

The moment ... *that* very instant ... is when you can

turn it around. Awareness is suddenly yours. You know what you are doing. And because you have learned that all humans make mistakes, you *won't* hate yourself for failing. Instead, you will tell yourself, "I'm going to finish this mouthful and then I will put my fork down and walk out of the room."

Saying it out loud is even more effective.

It's no different than the promises you have been making not to eat at certain hours of the day. *A binge is controllable behavior.*

Any time you stop, it's over, and that's that.

What is most destructive about a binge is not merely the uncontrolled eating. It's also excuse we have have that once we binge, there's no point in continuing with the diet.

People who binge think the contest lost. The effort has gone down the drain.

Nonsense! You didn't get fat overnight. So one binge —or even two or three binges—will not cause you to regain all the weight that you have lost. A binge is just an instance of being out of control. And now you know that you *can* get the control back.

Here's how I handle it.

The other night I had a wonderful dinner which was loaded with foods I don't normally eat. I ate and ate. I drank too. Lots of wine. Even as I ate I felt the waistband of my skirt tightening.

The next morning I couldn't decide whether I should or should not get on the scale. As I've described before, sometimes it helps and sometimes it definitely does not.

That morning, before I got on the scale I made up my mind that whatever the number, I'd make it work for me.

Sometimes I pick a figure that even I know can't be possible. After all, it's not really possible for me to have eaten that particular dinner and have gained ten pounds. But just for that moment I pretend that when I step on the scale it wil be ten pounds that I've added to my normal weight.

When I weighed myself the three pounds were within acceptable limits.

More often than not I would recommend *not* weighing yourself. Wait until the following morning, or even the day after that. The thinking in this case is, "What can the scale tell me that I don't know?" You know you ate too much, so it may only depress you and cause you to continue eating. Best to wait until you know the news will be good.

What was my next step?

I went to my wardrobe and decided that it was important for me to be aware of how it felt carrying around those pounds. That meant I put on a very tight pair of pants, so I couldn't forget the effort it would take to hook the waist. When I sat, I was uncomfortable. You probably have a pair of pants like that.

Sometimes I decide to wear something very loose fitting. I do that when I feel that wearing tight clothing is going to make me feel miserable and only cause me to feel sorry for myself and perhaps keep me bingeing. You learn quickly enough which path to follow. That's part of being honest with yourself.

At these moments my desire is to make myself aware that I need to regain control of my eating.

The next step is to plan that day's menu immediately. Make it a challenge—but one you know you will succeed with. Tell your spouse or friends that you would like their help that day because you want to get back on the reducing track.

Try to get involved in an activity that takes you away from food. Make a deliberate plan and stick to it. If you like to use your hands, pick up your knitting. Or start sanding that old paint-stained table you've been meaning to. If your hands are busy working, they won't be available to feed your face. You'll feel pleased with yourself and that will have only positive effects.

Try to be with people. Being alone may encourage overeating. There's safety in numbers.

Whatever you do, don't wait until tomorow. Because one day of control can probably undo most of the damage you think you've done.

It will also prepare you for other moments when you may binge again. Prepare you in the sense that you will have proved to yourself that you *can* get the control back. That way, when you recognize that "I'm doing it again" eating, you'll also be able to say, "I can take care of it."

Most of all, don't chastise yourself. Accept your behavior as that of a human with human frailties and step back onto the path you strayed from.

A binge is over the second *you* decide it is.

Your excess weight will continue to come off.

Bingeing frequently gives you a distorted sense of

how much you actually have consumed. You feel blown up. But once you gain control you will give your body a chance to empty itself of that bloat. In a day or two, or three, when you get on that scale you may be delighted to discover that you haven't done *that* much damage.

INTERMISSION EXERCISE

The next time you find yourself eating out of control, remember that you can stop it. Promise yourself *now* that you will gain control. The moment you say to yourself, "It's over," is the moment that your binge will end.

The Pleasures
of Being Thin

It's *great* being thin! I love it when people are astonished when I tell them that I used to be fat. I remember how I used to look enviously at thin people. Now I'm one of them!

Obesity is an illness that leaves no scar once you have recovered. Nobody can tell you used to be fat unless you let them in on your secret.

Being thin helps to keep you thin. When you start getting postive feedback from your friends and from your mirror you will like what you see and want to keep yourself that way.

At this point you have learned many ways to get thin. You also know how to stay that way. Life can be pleasure-full when *you* take control.

I used to be a believer in luck, both good and bad. Then I started to observe that "good luck" seems to come to certain people again and again while "bad luck" tags along behind others with frequency.

I can't promise that being thin is going to change your luck. I can tell you that it changed mine. I feel so good about myself that pleasant things happen to me all the time. When you become thin and stay thin and realize you did it for yourself and you know you did it because you care about yourself, don't be surprised if the quality of your life improves. The changes reflect your much improved self-esteem.

You can do that, or you can play house with every new diet that comes along, lose some weight and then gain it back. That way you can continue to make your contribution to the hundreds of millions of dollars spent yearly by dieters.

A friend asked me what my gimmick was. What's the trick in getting thin? And more important, what's the trick in staying thin?

I asked him if he was listening carefully because I was about to let him in on the secret. As he bent forward so as not to miss a word I told him softly what he already knew. The secret is that there is no secret. The secret is that if you're fat, *you know what you have to do.*

However, I short-changed him. I gave him only half an answer. There is indeed a "secret" and it is so sound that you'll never find it in diet books, diet articles in newspapers and magazines or ads for diet products.

I shall share this secret with you shortly.

This book is for all of you who have gimmicked yourselves to the hilt. It's for those of you who have closets full of bran left over from the high-fiber approach to

getting thin. It's for you, too, who have half-empty
containers of liquid protein, crowded out by partially
used tins of powdered protein.

This book is for all of you who have squirreled away
diet pills from assorted prescriptions of those "emergency" times when you need help over that plateau
period.

And let's not overlook those who have bowed to receive shots of HCG; or who have carried bags of spinach
leaves for the Scarsdale plan; or others who go in and
out of spas or fat farms.

This book is for all of you who are ready to admit that
no matter how many ways you have reduced, you have
never managed to keep your weight off.

Most of all, this book is for those who want to devote
their lives to the pleasures that eating can offer. If there
is a gimmick in my way of staying thin it is in my
determination not to eat any food that isn't going to
give me pleasure. And, even more, to never miss those
foods that do.

Most of those who stay fat believe they must satisfy
their appetite drives immediately. Those of us who stay
thin satisfy appetite too—but we are in control of when
we eat. Yes, it involves adopting a mature attitude and
sense of responsibility. But the gratification of taking
that responsibility is nothing less than terrific.

I'm not fat and I don't miss any good foods. Ironically,
I often eat more—even in quantity—than I did when I
was fat. Planning when and what you are going to eat
is the method. It's exciting to have control over your

food. You can stop thinking about dieting when you
know in advance that you have a satisfying menu ahead
of you.

When you are thin you'll get a genuine kick when
people watch as you consume food with a hearty appetite and wonder "How does she (or he) do it and
stay thin?"

Okay, Carole, you've told us all of that. But what is
the ulitmate way to get it off and keep it off?

You've waited a long time. There is a wonderfully
sound way to lose weight.

Once while attending the International Book Fair in
Frankfurt, Germany, a friend and I were having dinner.
Roger Price, the humorist who created Droodles and
Mad Libs, came along and sat with us. He watched
intensely while I ate.

The next day he made his confession.

It seems he hadn't been particularly hungry and so
didn't want to order any of the overpriced food. Looking
at my slim figure, Roger assumed that I'd never finish
the food on my plate. He'd eat my leftovers, and thus
fill his stomach and save an easy twenty dollars.

You can imagine his surprise to see me consume
everything, with obvious enjoyment.

When he told me the next afternoon how my appetite
had foiled his plans, he asked, "How can you eat that
much food and stay as thin as you are? You must be
naturally thin!"

One comment like that makes it all worth while.

When it was announced to the book trade that I was
writing this book, I found that I had indeed opened

myself up in the way I knew would be necessary in order for me to be able to help others to lose weight.

Once you're thin, do you really want to tell people you were fat? You can see the eyes measuring you, trying to imagine how you looked some forty-five pounds heavier.

But if my success in staying thin inspires you, it's added pleasure for both of us!

Few of us want to be, but many of us are fat.

But *some* of us aren't anymore! Since you can't tell merely looking at people you never know how many people have successfully reduced. When I researched this book I asked thin people if they'd ever had a weight problem.

I met a number of men and women who told me that they had been heavy. Without execption these were people who decided that they liked themselves thin and that it was worth the planning and trading off involved to stay that way. Not surprising (to me) is the fact that they were people who eat well and obviously enjoy food. If they can do it and I can do it you can do it too.

And now I'm going to give you the sure-fire way. It is so simple, so safe and so sound that you're going to wonder why *you* never thought of it before!

Toward a
Happy En— Beginning!

A good friend of mine who had been dreaming for more than twenty years about waking up thin made this amazing-to-him discovery. After two decades of wishing himself thin overnight, he now understands not only that it can't happen, but that if it did, the thinness would be temporary.

He had tried everything. He was a veteran of every kind of crash diet, starvation diet, foodless water fast, and pill swallowing, injection-enduring approach to discarding extra pounds.

He knew that it no longer mattered whether the "blame" lay with his mother, his bad habits, or his sugar blues.

What did matter was that, logically, he had come to understand that the extra pounds were his own responsibility; that no one held a pistol to his head to make him eat food and that there were certain truisms about "keeping it off" that none of the above dietary approaches contained.

His new found rule? "If it isn't natural, it won't endure."

In other words, any approach to weight loss that ends at some point will leave you as you were before. The only truly success-insured "diet" is one that you can live with for the rest of your life.

It sounds so simple, doesn't it?

He also learned the sad, scientifically-proved fact that weight lost rapidly will return rapidly.

His "new" approach to reducing was to *limit his weight* loss to a pound and a half a week.

He no longer weighs himself every day. He only allows himself to step on the scale once a week. That way he can compensate one day for the extra calories he may have eaten the previous evening.

He has chosen an extremely realistic approach towards reducing, *and it works beautifully!* He still has a great deal of weight to lose. However, he no longer is impatient because he isn't thin immediately. He loses his quota of pounds each week—every week.

He has a goal chart that he fills in faithfully.

If he loses less than a pound and a half, he goes on a one-day semi-fast. If he loses more than a pound and a half in any week, he considers it a bonus, but he manages to not be unrealistic about his plan. He has accepted the responsibility for making himself heavy and now he accepts the responsibility for making himself thin.

What he is doing is so sound that sometimes he feels he has invented the wheel. Nothing! He used to want to lose ten or fifteen pounds a week. And sometimes he did—then put them all back on again.

But this pound-and-a-half is magic. He isn't putting his body into shock. He isn't depriving himself of food.

What he is doing is slowly but perceptibly changing the way he thinks about food and acts about food.

When he has reached "goal" he won't have to make a drastic adjustment in his eating. He has gradually changed his eating habits. And these will be his habits forever.

As I write this he has been on his program for four months. He has lost twenty-seven pounds. On crash diets he lost that in a month. *But this weight he is likely to keep off forever.*

He can congratulate himself as he succeeds. For the first time in years he's actually *enjoying* dieting. He has the pleasure of watching the pounds go off, gradually, but regularly.

This is the concept I want you to try: Weight loss slowly but intelligently, a day at a time, but measured by the week. If you fall into the pits, you have the opportunity to jump out immediately and recover before the week ends.

Believe me when I tell you that lasting weight loss is married to time. Radical changes in your eating habits or sudden large weight losses are temporary for they're almost impossible to sustain.

Plan for a year. Assure yourself that "Next year at

this time I am going to be thin." Remember that woman I told you about who announced to her husband that she was going to enter college at the age of 50? When her husband tried to discourage her by saying that by the time she finished her degree she would be 54, she responded, "I'm going to be 54 in four years anyway, so I may as well be 54 *with* a college degree."

Losing weight at this rate will also enable your body to accustom itself naturally to the slow but steady change. You don't need a crash diet to lose at this pace. As a matter of fact, at first you hardly have to "diet" at all. You can probably just pick a couple of foods to cut out or cut down, and, presto, four pounds gone that first month.

A psychiatrist I know insists that this gradual way is the *only* way she knows that people lost weight *and kept it off!*

I want you to try it. Embark on the gradual approach I have just described.

Don't fall into the trap of believing you must lose a massive number of pounds in a short period of time. You're not in a race. You're embracing a positive and effective way to change your weight even as you change your eating style.

Set your own goals, both in number of pounds to lose and the length of time you'll take to lose them.

The time factor is not the critical ingredient. A pound a week? Why, that's fifty-two pounds a year—with almost no sacrifice and with its own built-in you've-taken-control-of-your-eating-so-you'll-keep-it-off insurance!

What *is* important is that you get thin *and stay thin.*

Naturally. Comfortably. And in your own way, eating the foods you like and liking the you that you're re-shaping.

Many psychiatrists, nutritionists and behavior modification specialists agree that this is the best of all possible methods.

Try it. It works wonderfully well. And one of these days you too can say, "I was once fat but I'll never be fat again!"

Good luck to you!

Bibliography

Beach, Nancy. "Variety: The Spice of a Well-Balanced Diet." *The New York Times Magazine*, January 28, 1979.

Berland, Theodore. "The Fat Chance Diet." *Politics Today*, March/April, 1978.

Bilgore, Ellen. "Losing Weight Successfully." *Vogue*, December, 1979.

Blackburn, G. L., M.D. "Dr. Blackburn's Calorie-Controlled Weight-Loss Program." *Family Circle*, November 20, 1979.

Bricklin, Mark. *Lose Weight Naturally: "Prevention" Magazine's No-Diet, No-Willpower Method.* Rodale Press, 1979.

Brody, Jane E. "Researchers Challenge Old Theories on Obesity." *The New York Times*, February 20, 1979.

Cohen, Toby. "Why Diets Don't Work." *New York Magazine*, May 21, 1979.

Danowski, T. S., Clare, D. W., Nolan, S., Stephan, T., Schmitt, T., Ahmad, U., and Fisher, E. R. "Prospective Study of Jejunoileal Bypass in Obesity." *Obesity/Bariatric Medicine*, vol. 5, no. 2, 1976.

Dufty, William, *Sugar Blues*. Chilton, 1975.

Dullea, George. "The Scarsdale Diet: If It's Friday, It Must Be Spinach and Cheese." *The New York Times,* July 7, 1978.

Eden, Alvin, N., M.D. "How Safe Is the Scarsdale Diet?" *Family Weekly,* December 3, 1978.

Elting, Melvin L., and Isenberg, Seymour. *You Can Be Fat Free Forever*. St. Martin's Press, 1974.

Geis, Jon H., Ph.D. *The Psychology of Dieting*. The Institute for Rational Living, N.Y.

Hafen, Brent Q. *Overweight and Obesity: Causes, Fallacies, Treatment*. Brigham Young University, 1975.

Headley, Lee, Ph.D. *People Around You Can Make You Fat*. Popular Library, 1979.

"How to Lose Weight Without Hunger." *Harper's Bazaar,* January, 1966.

Kopkind, Andrew. "The Age of Obesity." *Politics Today,* March/April, 1978.

Linn, Robert, with Stuart, Sandra Lee. *The Last Chance Diet*. Lyle Stuart, 1976.

"Making It." *Us* Magazine, August 21, 1979.

Mazzanti, Deborah Szekely. *Secrets of the Golden Door*. Bantam Books, 1979.

Nagler, Willibald E., M.D., "The Cellulite Myth." *Vogue,* August, 1979.

Pearson, Leonard, Ph.D., and Pearson, Lillian R., M.S.W. *The Psychologist's Eat-Anything Diet*. Peter Wyden, 1973.

Reuben, David, M.D. *Everything You Always Wanted to Know About Nutrition*. Avon Books, 1979.

Robertson, Donald S., M.D. *Obesity/Bariatrc Medicine,* vol. 8, no. 1, 1979.

Simeons, A. T. W., M.D. *Pounds and Inches (A New Approach to Obesity)*. Arti Grafiche Scalia, Rome, 1972.

Stillman, Irwin M., M.D., and Baker, Samm Sinclair. *The*

Doctor's Quick Weight Loss Diet. Prentice-Hall, 1967.

Tarnower, Herman, M.D., and Baker, Samm Sinclair. *The Complete Scarsdale Medical Diet.* Bantam Books, 1980.

"The Truth About the 25 Most Common Weight Control Myths." *Good Housekeeping* Magazine, November, 1972.

Tyson, Mary C., M.D., and Tyson, Robert, Ph.D. *The Psychology of Successful Weight Control.* Nelson-Hall Company, 1974.

Wechsler, H. L. "Vitamin Deficiency and Bypass Surgery." Also "Malnutrition and Bypass Surgery." *Obesity/Bariatric Medicine,* vol. 8, no. 6, 1979.

"What's All This Talk About Fiber?" *Redbook* Magazine, January, 1977.